23 WAYS
TO A
HAPPIER
LIFE

KAVITA BASI

Advance praise for 23 Ways to a Happier Life

"Brain Aneurysm survivor, Kavita Basi, is candid, funny, and motivational as she talks about turning a shattering life experience into a recipe for a positive lifestyle. Her commitment to giving back to the brain aneurysm community by sharing her personal experiences and approach to every day as a second chance continues to inspire all of us, especially those touched by this devastating disease. We are beyond proud to have Kavita as our supporter and Ambassador."

Erin Kreszl, Executive Director of The Bee Foundation for Brain Aneurysm Prevention

Published 6th May 2022
Printed in the United Kingdom
ISBN: 978-1-7396737-0-3 paperback
ISBN: 978-1-7396737-1-0 hardback
ISBN: 978-1-7396737-2-7 kindle (e-book)
ISBN: 978-1-7396737-3-4 audiobook

For information :
www.kavitabasi.com
Instagram @kavita_basi
FB @KavitaBasiroom23
Twitter @KavitaBasi
Youtube @Kavita Basi
Kavita Basi publishing
Interior design by Kavita Basi & Artful Editor L.A.
Illustrations by Eva Stibbe Nunney

I dedicate this book to my two children Jasmine and Jay and of course my little Brandi, whom I love with all my heart, they are the reason I am continuing to experience a better, more happier way of life.

CONTENTS

'A Simple Life,
Take out the complications
and see the
Happiness'

KAVITA BASI

AUTHORS NOTE

The stories I am sharing here are real life events that have happened to me post Brain-Haemorrhage and I share these with some of my favourite quotes that have had a huge effect on my state of mind, aswell as giving me an understanding of the Art of Happiness. My illustrations show the fun side of my personality and give visuals to those that prefer to grasp information this way due to Neuro conditions. Please check out the tips and enjoy these small moments of joy.

You must be the change you wish to see in the world.

—Mahatma Gandhi

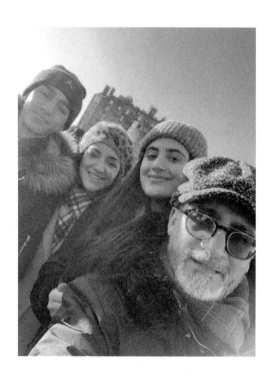

INTRODUCTION

December 2020

I'M POST FIVE and a half years after my subarachnoid brain hemorrhage (SAH) in March 2015, and all I think about is how grateful I am to be here. I'm alive and I will be okay! I can see that I have been given a second chance in life to be with my family, so I want to hold and cherish every single moment I have.

I'm a different person—yes, that's how I feel. I still don't know exactly what happened during my unconscious state in the hospital and during the weeks of memory loss I incurred. Did I lose the person I was and come out as someone else? It's a complete mystery to me. I still have some of the old Kavita's personality and physically look the same, but both my daughter, Jasmine, and husband, Deepak, constantly remind me that I am somewhat different. In Deepak's words, 'You look like Kavita, sound like Kavita, but you are someone else, and those eighteen years that we have had together are now being spent with a different person, and I have to adjust—it's hard.' Jasmine says that I have been born again and come back into the family in a new life. Listening to this just makes me wonder. It is all quite a mystery, but I have now left it to the Universe.

I feel like me, but I also have this small doubt that I'm not the same person that went into hospital late that evening on the 17th

March, fighting for her life, and this can feel a little sad. It can upset me, as I have this feeling that I have lost someone, like when I lost my father years ago—I have lost me, and for this I have needed to grieve. However, it has also given me a reason to celebrate and take hold of the life I have been given, and I don't want to waste a single moment. Enjoy each day and be in the present moment is how I live now.

I want to share some of my experiences on the road to recovery over the past few years that have helped me towards living a fuller, happier life. I hope, through reading this book, you can also enjoy your moments positively, cherish them and be happier, no matter what the circumstances. Whether it's emotional, mental, physical or financial, we all go through our ups and downs, but celebrating and embracing the ups keep the positive energy going, which can grant some much-needed hope and happiness. To experience the happiness in life, you have to experience the difficulties too. It's inevitable, so it can help to embrace what is to come for you.

This book is filled with some of my favourite positive-energy quotes. Some are from great, inspirational people, these are quotes that I love and live by. They help motivate me, and I often share them on my social media so others may be motivated too. The short stories of my experiences through the last few years and what I have learnt from them give me the positivity I live by today. My Neuropsychologist explained to me that recovery is an ongoing process. I keep this in my mind and continue to strive. It motivates me to be better, do better and live better.

Please note : Even though there are timelines mentioned within each chapter, the short stories are not in a chronological sequence of events. The purpose for this is because I would like this to be a keepsake book and for you to randomly choose a story that you wish to learn more of at any given time.

Finally, I decided to add quick response (QR) codes to my book to bring together my love of forecasting and interactive design and my desire to reach and hold the interest of future generations and of people recovering from brain trauma. Visual media has played a large role in my recovery. I haven't been able to read in the same way since the onset of my illness. My doctor says this is typical for people who have suffered brain injuries. My hope is that by offering this interactive approach to the book, readers may have a more layered experience of my stories. To download a QR code scanner, just visit the app store on your smartphone or try the camera on your mobile device.

Would love to connect with you!

If you want a little motivation or like to get
some positive vibes, please follow me on

Instagram @kavita_basi

Twitter @KavitaBasi

Facebook @KavitaBasiroom23

Otherwise, you can email me or follow my blog on
www.kavitabasi.com.

#HopeAndHappiness #Recovery
#DoingGoodLivingBetter #ANewMe

Barcode www.kavitabasi.com

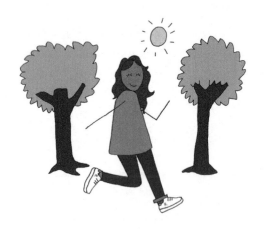

CHAPTER 1

Every day is a new beginning.
Take a deep breath, smile and start again.

—AUTHOR UNKNOWN

Walking is good for you

IT'S AUGUST 2019, and sitting here thinking about what I would like to share is daunting, but my reason for doing so is that sharing my experiences could make a difference that improves someone else's life. I always have so much information going on inside my head, and now that I have no filter, I just say and do what I'm thinking at the time. It's refreshing to new people I meet, but for my family, it's an absolute pain to deal with, as they have to listen and adjust to this new me—and here she goes again! This is how I am. I feel I give my family an adventure each time we start something new. Life is supposed to be an experience filled with lots of adventures, right?

Now, walking every day is one of the best forms of therapy I have encountered since my illness. It isn't too strenuous, it's easy to manage the time and, rain or shine, I do it. I walk because it makes me feel better. I feel amazing because not only will I lose a few calories on the way, but my head is clear of all the junk it seems to carry around constantly. Walking has improved my mental health and general well-being. After a walk, I am refreshed and ready to take on anything in my head, although physically, it exhausts me! I always need to have a good rest after my walk as I just don't have the same energy I used to before the hemorrhage. Walking also gives me some silence—one of the side effects I have endured is high anxiety, so I need calm to help focus my mind.

I go for a brisk, short walk around my hometown, and even that feels like an adventure to me. I harness up Brandi, my puppy, and get all her things together and grab a family member—one of my children or my husband—to tag along with me. I put my sweatshirt on—in the north of England, there is always a chance of rain—and then I step out into the full abundance of nature! I absolutely love the feeling of being outside; it is one of the things that has helped my recovery process in terms of exercise and clearing my thoughts to reduce my high anxiety. Nobody else understands this. To my family, it sometimes becomes another chore they have to do. They wouldn't ever let me go alone because of the worry that I may have a seizure or fall, but they do see the benefits it has on me later. Walking makes me happy, and this happiness transfers to everyone around me. If this is what a simple task can do, then why not embrace it? Walking does not need an abundance of money or pressure behind it. It's a simple way of improving well-being, and all you need is to put aside a little time to ensure you get the best out of this wonderful experience.

When I returned to work in October 2015, I found it extremely hard to focus at times and needed some time out. So during my lunch break, I made a point of walking outside around the perimeter of my work building. It would keep me focused and help with my workday when everything was getting to be too much for me. I would return to my desk smiling, relieved of all pressure and ready to continue my work. This was the best thing I ever started—I could see the benefits of it almost instantly.

I added a walk after dinner in the evening, and then another in the morning. Maybe it was asking too much of my family to join in every time, but I really needed my walks and fresh air to help me, so that's when I decided I needed a different sort of companion other than my husband. Due to my previous health scare, I wasn't allowed to walk alone, as my family was always worried that something might happen again. They just wanted me safe, and I understood. So we decided on getting a puppy—Brandi!

It's the bank holiday, August 2019, and we are on our way to the beautiful landscape of the Lake District, which is situated around ninety-five miles north of Manchester. It's not a huge distance to be transported to a geographical wilderness of rolling mountains with beautiful clear lakes, trickling streams and adventurous walking trails. It is a stunning part of the United Kingdom that is a must-see for all visitors.

Deepak, Jasmine, my son, Jay, and I packed the car with blankets, towels, a few snacks and plenty of water bottles. Even Brandi had a little rucksack packed with her toys and treats! We were all ready for our little adventure. I filmed the scenic countryside and wildlife along the way while listening to my kids' playlist and trying to understand their modern music choices. It was so much fun, and I was looking forward to meeting up with our friends and their families to enjoy a rare day of warm British summer.

After struggling to park the car in a very busy tourist area, we eventually got settled, met everyone and started our trek at the edge of Grasmere Forest. Grasmere is a village and tourist destination in the centre of the Lake District. It takes its name from the adjacent lake. It has associations with the Lake Poets— William Wordsworth lived in Grasmere for fourteen years and called it 'the loveliest spot that man hath ever found.'

Walking through the trees, following the small wooden signposts leading the way into the forest reminded me of something out of *The Wind in the Willows*. Brandi was so excited, scuffling full speed ahead, sniffing each part of the woodland—this was a new playground of exploration for her. She started to jump around to get ahead so she could see more of this enchanting place. We hopped over graveled footpaths where streams were crossing, walked uphill through turns and twists in the forest, and then we arrived at the most beautiful open area, a pebbled beach surrounding a huge, glistening, crystal-blue lake. This spectacular view reminded me of the trips I had taken previously to Lake Garda in Italy, and to see this literally on our doorstep was just breathtaking. That was it—the weather was so warm that it encouraged all the children and some of the dads to strip down and jump into the lake. Brandi joined them. It was so lovely to see this simple enjoyment. The only technology being used was my phone to capture some of the moments in photos.

After drying off and taking a moment to rest, we were off again to climb one of the small mountains, or you could have called it a very large hill. The luscious, tall greenery around us teamed with the heat of the day made it feel like we were in some tea-farming district in the middle of Bali. One of our friends was carrying their little baby tightly, the others were holding the hands of their young ones, helping them over some of the rocky paths. Deepak was busy catching up on football chat with his friend, and Jay was way ahead exploring the rocks and cliffs and climbing up some of the surrounding areas. It was lovely to see Jasmine chatting to my friend, expressing her excitement about leaving home to start university. I, on the other hand, was focused on the present, taking it all in and just admiring how much I was enjoying this walk☺.

After what seemed like a trek, we reached the top, and to my surprise, we were faced with a stepping-stone effect of large flat stones over a small lake that led into a mammoth cave. Another amazing sight that I was just not expecting. Like a small, inquisitive child, I immediately started to step across the stones, wanting to see more of this mysterious cave. It was extraordinary that we had all of this area to explore around us and I had never been, in all the forty-three years I had lived in my home country, but at least I was there now!

This had to be at the top of my list of best days post hemorrhage. I do believe, though, that my mindset has a lot to do with how much I actually enjoy my life experiences. Walking has a great positive effect on me. The sounds of nature, smell of leaves and flowers, the feel of a slight breeze against my skin all make a huge difference to my well-being and happiness. It could do the same to yours. It is most definitely my favourite time of the day!

5 things you can do for a happy walk:

1. Catch up on your favourite playlist or audiobook, but for health and safety, don't turn the volume too loud.

2. Go with a child, sibling or parent for some family one-on-one time! Face-to-face attention will surely help love grow.

3. Ask a friend to join you, and catch up on what they have been doing. It's nice to use your time valuably.

4. Grab a lovely hot drink in a flask to enjoy on your walk. Why not try a flower tea or almond milk matcha latte?

5. Join a walking club in your area. Enquire in your local meet-up, social club or Facebook groups. You could meet some new friends that love walking too!

Barcode Grasmere Lake District

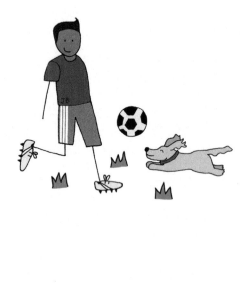

CHAPTER 2

**You get in life what you have
the courage to ask for.**

—OPRAH WINFREY

I want a puppy! March 2019

MY SON, JAY, had been mithering us for as long as I could remember about wanting a dog. We thought it was a phase, as all children go through, but this phase did not seem to pass. I absolutely love dogs and had a couple of them in my youth. Unfortunately, Jasmine and Deepak were both petrified of them, and Deepak's parents, who live with us, were not really dog lovers—I think the term they used was that they were allergic! This just wasn't going to happen in the near future. I then thought about my walking sessions, where I required a companion, and it seemed like this could be an option for me and a way to lessen the burden on my family. But having a puppy is like looking after a child—the care, time, grooming and attention are all part of the package. It's 100 percent correct when people say it isn't just a trophy. Dogs need attention and care as much as we do, so it was going to be a huge commitment for us all if we decided to go through with it.

I put it off for quite some time, and on his eighth birthday, we got Jay two Russian tortoises in a large tank with some small ornaments. This was going to be our starting point to see how Jay would be around his own pets. We already had a fish tank full of various tropical species that only I or Deepak's mum would feed each day. The novelty does wear off, so I had to try another test. There were a couple of reasons for getting the tortoises. I wanted to reward him by giving him the opportunity to have pets that he could interact with so he could gain some understanding on what was involved in their routines. It would also give us the confidence that he could take on more responsibility. In the beginning, he would do everything: feed them, bathe them, let them out in the garden when it was warm. They originated in a desert habitat, so for a number of hours each day, they had to be kept under a solar lamp or in direct sunlight. Well, as with any pet, the novelty soon fizzled.

I could see that he probably needed a pet that could interact with him more and that he could teach tricks to, play football or run with—he loves his sports. We waited another four years, and this time, it was so exciting. We did mounds of research beforehand, as well as checking with breeders through an accredited site, The Kennel Club UK, to ensure we were getting a puppy that suited our lifestyle and would fit in with our family. The excuses from his father had run out, and now it was Jay's turn to seize his opportunity☺.

I remember the day we went to visit the litter of puppies. They were only a few days old. Jay was so excited, and I was too! They were so little, approximately hamster sized and had that newborn, farm-like smell. We looked at the whole litter, snuggled up together in soft blankets and the mum sitting nearby, licking them to check if they were okay. There were males and females, black, black with tan patches, and all tan. Jay selected this beautiful tan-coloured puppy with a lilac band collar and held it in his hand. It fit neatly in his palm. He had chosen a girl, and she was absolutely adorable!

We had to wait until she was three months old and ensure our home was fully dog-proofed before adopting her. But when the day finally arrived and we went to collect her, there were smiles and excitement all around. Jay held her next to him, wrapped up tightly, all the way home. I could not believe we were going to have a new addition to our family—this gorgeous working cocker spaniel called Brandi Basi.

It was a challenge, but only for the first few weeks—potty training, removing all the things that got chewed, covering furnishings, cleaning messes and hiding any shoes that we didn't want shredded. I also had Deepak's parents to consider; they were much older and set in their ways. But Brandi fit in like a dream, a ray of sunshine all around us—even Deepak. Jasmine also overcame her fear of dogs and quickly became one of the closest to Brandi. She even has her sitting in bed with her in the evenings whilst watching her programs. Brandi sits patiently as Jay intently does his homework, and she loves playing football in the garden, running back and forth across the goals to follow the ball. She is surprisingly obedient and calm in Deepak's presence. She gives unconditional love to us all. However, the best is that I now have my walking companion!

We are now two years on, and we love her more than ever. We do morning walks, evening walks and family walks on the weekend. This has changed our lifestyle—we experience more of the outdoors, and caring for another family member has brought us closer. It has also given both Jasmine and Jay some much-needed responsibility, not to mention a new friend. Mr Basi Senior—Deepak's dad—likes to take her out to play in the garden whilst he sits and relaxes with his cup of tea, and Mrs Basi Senior—Deepak's mum—has a night-time companion on the sofa whilst she catches up with her TV dramas. Brandi loves to get all prepped with her small treat bag—she knows that when the coats and bags are ready, she is about to start another adventure. But her absolute favourite thing is going somewhere in the car. She gets so excited to see where we will end up.

My anxiety has been considerably reduced by having Brandi

around, and when I have had a hard day at work, once I see her and spend a few minutes with this playful pup, my mind is filled with complete joy and happy thoughts. She has completely changed the atmosphere of our home, and I couldn't imagine life without her now. It has all been so worth it. The persistence of Jay and a little push from me led to one of the best decisions we have made. Brandi's little innocent face and long, floppy, crimped ears are too cute not to adore. She senses everyone's likes and dislikes and uses them to her advantage to win everyone over. This has increased the love in our household. Breakfast time, walking time, dinnertime are all centered around Brandi, and it is amazing!

5 things we love about Brandi:

1. Mellow to be around—Deepak
2. Removes all anxiety—Kavita
3. Playful puppy—Jasmine
4. My best friend—Jay
5. Our very cute family member—Mr and Mrs Basi Senior

Barcode Brandi running in the fields

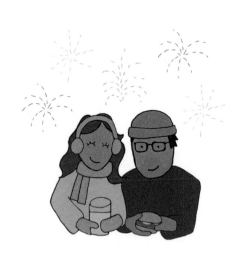

CHAPTER 3

Be happy in the moment, that's enough.
Each moment is all we need, not more.

—MOTHER TERESA

Guy Fawkes Night, November 2018
'REMEMBER, REMEMBER, THE fifth of November!' We all get excited to celebrate Bonfire Night, or Guy Fawkes Night. I've always loved Bonfire Night, but have you ever stopped to think what implications this can have for others that may have anxiety or hearing deficiencies? It must be a difficult time, not to mention the poor little pets that are frightened by the loud bursts and bangs continuing through the evening and late into the night.

I HAVE CHILDHOOD memories of going with my family—my two sisters, baby brother in a pram and my very excited parents—in the cold, crisp evening to a nearby school with a huge open field, all of us wrapped up warm with hats, gloves, scarves and big wellies, ready to watch this spectacular display that only happened once a year. We would get some warm popcorn, hot chocolate and other snacks to have whilst staring into the amazing, colourful lights in the sky. The best was the fascinating Catherine wheel that would go so fast it made your eyes go funny. I didn't ever want these wonderful family evenings to end. My father would even get us ice cream in the freezing cold weather on the way home, just to have that extra enjoyment! This is one of my happy memories of my late father that I now cherish.

Now it's a completely different situation. My children are older, so they're off to see the displays with their friends in groups. I tried to go to a nearby display, but after ten minutes, I couldn't handle the noise, and the pain in my ears was just dreadful. I used to love going with my family. It was a highlight for me to get all wrapped up to watch the array of lights and bump into neighbours and friends for some socialising while celebrating the history behind Guy Fawkes Night.

However, since my SAH, I have struggled with particular noises. It's only when I'm feeling overtired or if the sounds are very high pitched, then they cause immense pain in my ears—probably the same way they affect a dog. Because I also suffer from high anxiety—another side effect—when I'm in a very crowded place, I have an overwhelming sense of suffocation, and this can result in panic attacks. If I go, I need to be in a much wider space, and I have to wear earplugs. That way I can still enjoy the evening and not feel like I'm missing out on normal family activities. I'm far from normal, but I have learned to embrace this new, changed me, so I have a plan and I'm determined to try this new experience. I can still enjoy my evening—I just have to adapt now.

We all get ready with our outdoor attire, and I have my make-shift earplugs. My little puppy has to stay behind in a warm, safe room that blocks out the noise. She is snuggled up comfortably with Deepak's parents so she won't be alone. Jay is excited to meet his friends, and Jasmine makes her own plans to meet up with hers. My face is lit up, and I feel a sense of eagerness.

We walk towards the large football club venue situated between the Hale and Bowdon residential areas. It's close to our home, and as we wait patiently in the queue, I start to hear the crowds shouting and the fireworks. I put tissues inside my ears and instantly feel at ease. We are all given a wristband and a stamp on the top of our hands as we go through the small, gated pathway. As we enter, Jasmine spots her friends and starts to rush off with excitement. We ask her to keep Jay by her side and hand over some cash so that Jay can enjoy the rides and, of course, some sweet treats.

Deepak and I stay near the entrance—it's less crowded, and there is the added bonus of a great viewing platform. I look around at all the other families greeting their neighbours with handshakes and friends with hugs. Children are running around with excitement, holding small spinning-light toys they have just bought at the stalls. Fathers have their little ones sitting on their shoulders so they can see the displays. I can faintly hear the music playing from the fairground carousels nearby and the announcements giving the times for the next display to start.

The smell of smoking wood and candy floss combined with savoury treats is making me hungry. Deepak gets me a vegan burger and himself a beer, and we stand and watch. I look up and see each firework take off and explode into a burst of the most amazing colours. I haven't done this for a couple of years due to the extreme side effects—high anxiety, hearing issues with high-pitched or loud sounds, claustrophobia, headaches, short-term memory loss—I've endured after my illness. I learned to adapt to them over time, and this feels like the first time I have ever seen this creative display of light and vibrant colours in the sky. Truly spectacular. At the time, I couldn't explain to my family this moment I was experiencing, but they knew I was happy there with them, adapting to my new life—new me and new surroundings. Happy Guy Fawkes Day!

Adaptation is about having these new experiences and enjoying them as much or maybe even more than before. Let's be positive, adapt and enjoy each moment.

If you'd like to learn more about Guy Fawkes Day, the BBC

have done a great piece about the history behind it: *http://www.bbc.co.uk/history/people/guy_fawkes*

Barcode family picture

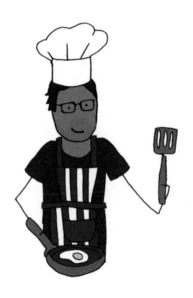

CHAPTER 4

Gratitude is the healthiest of all human emotions.

—ZIG ZIGLAR

Unconditional Love, February 2018

APPRECIATE YOUR UNCONDITIONAL love. I read in an article from one of my favourite authors—'The Rules of Love', by Richard Templar—that you always give your nearest and dearest (your partner, mother, siblings, children) the toughest time, only because you have that unconditional love for them. All your frustrations are also offloaded onto them, and you just can't help it!

So why not take a step back and see all the lovely things that they do for you? If a friend or stranger does something nice for you, it's natural to thank them and appreciate their kindness. So why not show the same appreciation to your loved ones? It's very easy to become used to them and start to take them for granted. Think about it—when did you say, 'Thank you for getting me that drink' or 'I appreciate your time on the walk with me'? Everyone loves a little gratitude. Even if you have spent a lifetime with them, it's so valuable.

I make a point of having a weekly family meeting and telling my husband and children all the helpful things they do to make my life easier since my illness, and it has made them do more! When I leave for work in the morning, my husband has my flask ready with herbal tea and the car warmed up. Once a week, my daughter prepares our family meal to help take the stress off me, and now I say that I really appreciate it. Those little things you say go a very long way, trust me.

I have suffered from extreme fatigue, short-term memory loss and high anxiety, and all these small acts of kindness from my close family have been so helpful, allowing me to lead as normal a life as possible. I know it will never be the same as it was before the SAH, so I always express my gratitude to my family. I now understand that even though it was me that went through the operations and difficulties in recovery and trauma, these things also affected my close family, and they have had to adjust too. Oh, I love them.

Our little puppy has this unconditional love too. We can actually learn from some of their behavioural attributes as humans. We just plough through life with lots of chores, things to do, work to complete, and sometimes we need to just reset our way of thinking and our actions, take a moment to appreciate the present and what's in front of us. Yes, it may take a little longer to complete the task in hand, but at least it will have been done with some appreciation.

I have the same ethics in the workplace—I always make a point of letting the team know that I value their input and appreciate their time. I know it's their job and they would do the task anyway, but I always like that other person to know how they have done. It boosts their morale too. It's how I treat my family. I have worked in some big corporate environments and seen the brutal shouting and bullying that happens between management and team members, and it's just not the right way to behave. If you give more love and express gratitude, you will definitely achieve more.

Love can be shown in so many ways; it doesn't have to be in words, or a letter, email, message or even a gift. It can be shown by giving your time and attention to those around you—these are priceless and sharing them will always give you a great sense of fulfilment as well as that unconditional love. I do this by calling my mother almost daily to check in to see if she's okay, listen to her tasks of the day, or programs she has been watching or her daily complaining about her back or sleep or general politics of what's happening in the world. She knows I'm here to listen and take some of the burden away. My husband also likes this attention, especially when telling me of his work issues. I just sit and listen and don't tell him about my problems—I'm giving my time to him. Why not share that time with someone who needs it, and in return feel that lovely fulfilment?

I don't have as much energy as I used to, and my husband is always doting over me, making me a cup of tea in the morning or making my brunch—eggs on toast. We had been married eighteen years when I became ill, and he had never been a cook at all, but it seems that now he has become a master chef in our home! I suppose he had no choice, but for me it shows that unconditional love: he is doing something completely out of his comfort zone to make my day feel easier. So, on a weekend when I'm a little more relaxed and have some energy, I always try and cook something that I know he will enjoy and appreciate. Or I sit with him while he watches old episodes of *Only Fools and Horses*, which I don't have any interest in, but I like to give him some company. I want him to feel that sense of gratitude from me too. This situation has increased our love for each other even further. This is the essence of being kind to one another. Kindness is key for that unconditional love.

Valentine's Day is a lovely time to share that love. It doesn't have to be with a partner—it can be your mother, father, a friend. Wouldn't it be great to just send them a little card to say how much you value them and show your unconditional love? I would like to share some details of why we celebrate Valentine's Day and why it's an important time to appreciate one another:

The Legend of St Valentine

Valentine was a priest who served during the third century in Rome. When Emperor Claudius II decided that single men made better soldiers than those with wives and families, he outlawed marriage for young men. Valentine, realizing the injustice of the decree, defied Claudius and continued to perform marriages for young lovers in secret. When Valentine's actions were discovered, Claudius ordered that he be put to death.

St Valentine, according to some sources, is actually two distinct historical characters who were said to have healed a child while imprisoned and executed by decapitation.

The history of Valentine's Day—and the story of its patron saint—is shrouded in mystery. We do know that February has long been celebrated as a month of romance, and that St Valentine's Day, as we know it today, contains vestiges of both Christian and ancient Roman tradition. (History.com)

For more information, please follow the link below:

History of Valentine's Day - Facts, Origins & Traditions - HISTORY

Whatever is written about how St Valentine started this wonderful tradition that we all celebrate today, one thing is for sure—it all started with love. So go home and say 'thank you' or 'I love you'. Or call a friend and tell them how much you value their friendship. Make someone happy on Valentine's Day—or any day—and show your unconditional love and appreciation. The tips below may be obvious, but we often don't realise how something so little can make such a huge difference to somebody's day.

5 ways to show a little appreciation:

1. Say thank you.
2. Give a hug.
3. Hold someone's hand.
4. Say 'I love you'.
5. Smile and show them how much they mean to you.

Barcode Deepak and Kavita, Maria Luisa Park

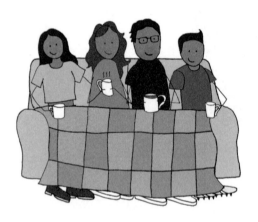

CHAPTER 5

When I was five years old, my mother always
told me that happiness was the key to life. When
I went to school, they asked me what I wanted
to be when I grew up. I wrote down happy. They
told me I didn't understand the assignment,
and I told them they didn't understand life.

—John Lennon

Love and happiness, December 2017

ALL YOU NEED is love and to show it. In turn, it will make you happy!
The December holidays are a festive time of the year that makes
everyone so busy! Buying gifts, arranging where to have Christmas
dinner, decorating the house and simply trying to make all things
perfect—especially for the children—on *the* special day. But at this
time, there is one important thing that can bring everyone together,
and that is a small token to show your love. I spent one Christmas
weekend with my side of the family up in the northeast of England,
seeing my mum, sisters, my brother, their spouses and their children, playing board games, eating and laughing together. It was so
much fun, and this has no monetary value at all—it just shows love

and happiness. It was effortless, incurred no expense and was a very simple way of making other people happy. We should all do it more often and show our appreciation of each other.

Since my father passed, I have found it important to have a great deal more quality time with my own family—Deepak, Jasmine and Jay. I have very fond and happy memories of my father and would want them to have the same once we leave them. Our evenings are spent playing board games, watching a movie together, snuggled up in our bed or getting a bunch of blankets and some hot chocolate and sitting in our lounge watching old videos of when the children were very young—they always like to watch themselves☺. These are my happy times, memories that, hopefully, they will pass on to their families when they move forward with their lives. Love and happiness are what makes life so fulfilling.

One year I made one of those 'homemade' wooden Christmas advent calendars. My son painted and decorated it, and then I had to fill in all the drawers, which traditionally hold a present or chocolate for each day. I did put in a few presents and chocolates, but most of the drawers were filled with happy little notes. 'Give someone you love a hug today' or 'Tell a friend what you like about them and make them happy'. I know you might think I'm being a bit mean by not giving him twenty-five chocolates, but I thought it was important because these small acts of kindness really add a little more love to the world. This Christmas, it would be lovely to do a good deed, meet or call your family and friends, tell them something that you like about them to make them happy. If you really want to go that extra mile, visit a neighbour that may not have any close relatives. Drop in for a cup of tea or invite them around for dinner. Visit a local homeless shelter and drop off some food or blankets or visit a local senior home and offer to help. There are so many ways to do this. The real meaning of this festive time is truly to show your love and make someone happy—and why not?

I never understood the true meaning of happiness until after my illness. It's as simple as sitting with my family and having dinner together, which puts a great big smile on my face. Or opening the bedroom curtains in the morning and seeing the sunshine—that makes me happy. Eating a bowl of rhubarb crumble and custard—oh, it gives me the best feeling. The key is to be happy with the simple things, and once you show them to the people around you, they will feel it too.

Go on, raise those endorphins!

5 ways to show your love to make someone happy this Christmas:

1. Express gratitude—tell someone how much you appreciate them.

2. Set aside time—give the gift of listening.

3. Be thoughtful with gifts—really understand the person and what is special about them.

4. Write a note—'I love you for a million reasons, and these are the top 3!'

5. Be forgiving—gently explain and then switch to a positive outlook.

Barcode Tavern on the Green, New York City

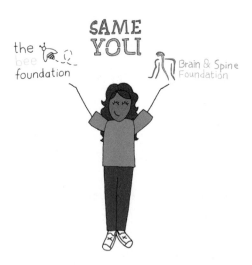

CHAPTER 6

**If you can do what you do best and be happy,
you are further along in life than most people.**

—Leonardo DiCaprio

It's a New Year! January 2019

It's New Year's Day! Yay! Let's take this opportunity to encourage others to help out☺. I will do my part by continuing my mission of raising awareness for neurological conditions through my speaking events and website. If you would like to be a part of this, please subscribe at *www.kavitabasi.com.* My website is a tool for me to share my experiences with the community. I write about some of my experiences after suffering my SAH. The stories involve my family, lifestyle, holidays and food! There are two other blogs linked to the site: Jasmine's, where she shares her love of fashion, politics and travel, and my sister Rajni's, who is not only in a high-powered job for an established law firm but absolutely loves to cook and create recipes for the family. Her creations are just divine. I also use this website to showcase my radio interviews, podcasts, books and other publications so that anyone that wants to know more about me can get a true sense of what I'm trying to do. I'm a Living Social Butterfly.

I am also a community ambassador for the Brain & Spine Foundation to continue fundraising and raise awareness for neuro conditions. If you'd like to support and help, please follow here: *https://www.brainandspine.org.uk/about-us/our-community-ambassadors/*. The Brain & Spine Foundation have been a support network for me and my family, and I enjoy being an ambassador for them, speaking and sharing their information—especially on social media—to help others. They give information for some of the 470 known neurological conditions, share articles in their booklets and on their website and also give great advice for patients, families and carers that need it. My time so far with them has been helpful for my own recovery and has prompted me to become not only their ambassador but also seek similar roles for The Bee Foundation in Philadelphia, USA, and SameYou in the UK.

The Bee Foundation—The mission of The Bee Foundation is to raise awareness of brain aneurysms and increase funding for innovative research that changes lives.

Meet Honey Bash Guest Speaker Kavita Basi - The Bee Foundation

SameYou.org—Their mission is to improve the neurorehabilitation process; it's also a great charity that reaches out to younger stroke survivors and families.

I share videoblogs through my YouTube channel to give visuals of what I went through, as visual media has played a big role in my recovery process. I now find it hard to read with the same capacity and can miss words and sentences as a result. And with short-term memory loss, it's easier for me to take in information from visuals, such as videos or pictures. To reach out to others in a similar position to me has been a great way to connect.

The release of my first book, *Room 23: Surviving a Brain Hemorrhage*, was one of my biggest achievements. This book shares my experiences after suffering a subarachnoid brain hemorrhage and my recovery process over a period of time to give the reader a sense of what happens when dealing with a neurological hidden illness. After sharing my video blogs, I felt that they didn't have enough reach to help others, so putting all my diary entries to use as a book seemed like the right thing to do. *Room 23* also helps to increase awareness of a condition that is part of a group of neurological illnesses that affect one in four people, so I decided to give back by donating 10 percent of the profits to the Brain & Spine Foundation so they can continue their vital work to help the neuro-affected community.

If you have purchased *Room 23*, I would love for you to post a photo with it on social media and tag me in! The Amazon link is here,

https://www.amazon.co.uk/Room-23-
Surviving-Brain-Hemorrhage/dp/1631524895/
*ref=mp_s_a_1_3?ie=UTF8&qid=1545029421&sr=8-3&pi=AC_SX236_*
SY340_QL65&keywords=room+23&dpPl=1&dpID=411TsxkSzSL&ref=plSrch,

Or go to the main page heading and follow the links for *Room 23*.

Through my work, I would like to use my knowledge and experience to make the right decisions for the growing fashion industry, especially on sustainable fashion. I want to create more products that are made in better, more ethical ways to reduce the fashion industry's polluting effects on our environment. I'm a big advocate of ethical fashion and making a difference in the industry.

In addition to my other roles, I don't want to forget to be the best role model I can for my children and a dedicated, loving wife. Even though I can't devote the same amount of time to my family as I used to, I want to spend the time I have with them, to focus on giving them the best of me. I have always believed in leading by your actions and example.

Finally, I'm trying to be the best version of me. Investing time in yourself is the best gift you can give—to yourself and those around you. If you want to read that great motivational book, then go ahead and do it. If you want to change your lifestyle for the better by eating healthier or doing some exercise, then go ahead. I promise you will feel goodness back in abundance! I wake up an hour early each morning, around five or six, and I spend this time investing in myself. The idea came from a book by Hal Elrod called *Miracle Morning*. It has been a great choice, as I can use my time in a very effective way and then focus on the things I need to when my household is up. My hour is usually spent listening to an audiobook, drawing, painting or just meditating. If you can try this, believe me, you won't go back—it's the best thing I've ever started.

Why not be the best version of you? You can also be part of helping others by checking out my blog, books and website. Please share, and let's spread the love and positive vibes! You can check out my publications that have been in newspapers, magazines, radio and other media. Please see link here: *https://www.kavitabasi.com/publications-1*. This has all happened because I have followed my true mission: to spread love and happiness☺.

#HappyNewYear2019 #MissionToHelpOthers #Room23
#PositiveAffirmations #PositiveVibes #RaisingAwareness
#BrainAndSpine #NeurologicalConditions #MyStory #Sustainability
#Mummy #LoveFamily #IAmHere #KavitaBasi

Barcode Kavita New Year'sDay

Barcode Waterstones book signing

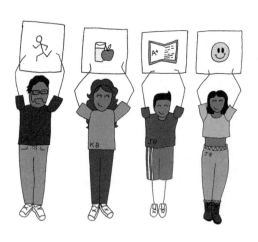

CHAPTER 7

**Every morning we are born again. What
we do today is what matters most.**

—Jack Kornfield

Cleanse Your Life, 2018

Cleanse your life! It's the New Year! It's our chance to start with a
clean slate and really focus on what's important. As well as detoxing
to cleanse our bodies, why not also cleanse our life? Imagine you
wanted to start your life all over again—what would you do? What
things do you love to spend time doing that you don't have time
for anymore? What makes you who you are and nourishes your
personality? If your life is black and white, let's try and bring some
colour back into it!

We went out for a family meal on New Year's Day, as it was
my husband's birthday—I know, more presents! But that year we
decided to do things a little differently. I took a small pad of paper
and four pens for a challenge during dinner. Everyone has resolu-
tions, and sometimes it's difficult to get them all done, so I asked
everyone to write just four New Year's goals that they wanted to
achieve and why. Then they folded the paper and passed it to the

family member on their left, who then read it out to the rest of us. It was so much fun and very interesting. Whilst reading each other's goals, we quickly realised that they all had common themes:

1. Achieving a milestone event, like participating in a run or marathon

2. Keeping healthy, like drinking more water or exercising

3. Emotions, like being happier

4. Personal goals, like doing well in school

I feel that I have been given a blank canvas in life—a second chance. I will take this opportunity to renew myself, go back to who I used to be as a child or teenager before life situations changed me. I love painting, I love music, and I love being social and learning. I ensure that each day contains a few minutes of doing things I like so that I can enjoy these moments.

My health is my wealth. Yoga and meditation keep me going and help me focus on the goals I want to achieve. Starting my day with just fifteen minutes of these as a way to ground myself has made a huge shift in achieving my goals. If you haven't tried it, I would encourage it—my life feels cleansed, focused and happy.

Another personal favourite of mine is creating a vision board. If there is something you really want to achieve in your life this year, this month, whenever, cut some photos out of magazines, draw some images, or put together some things you like in your home or room that you enjoy looking at to give you that positive inspiration. This is the start of your vision board, which can give you some focus on what you want to achieve in your life. It was one of the best things I did after returning from hospital—I needed to focus on some positive images that really encompassed my being to give me a sense of purpose.

Once these goals are posted on your vision board or written on a list, the challenging part is to actually follow through. I have told my family to keep the list of goals on their bedside table or stick it on a wall so that when they wake up every morning, it's the first thing they see. To make sure you are committed to your New Year challenges, it's important to keep looking at them, as they can be easily forgotten, especially after deciding on them on that day. Another way to keep your goals in constant check is to put them on your screen saver on your phone or computer. We want to visualise these daily! And give yourself a timeline for each goal so it isn't left on the back burner; otherwise, it will be a case of 'I will just do that another time.' So let's do this!

5 ways to stay on track with your New Year's goals:

1. Post your list where you'll see it first thing in the morning.

2. Make it a screen saver on your phone or computer so you're reminded throughout the day.

3. Set a deadline or a series of milestones to reach by a certain date.

4. Make yourself accountable! Tell your friends and family—you might be able to help them out with their goals.

5. Track your progress on an app or just a sheet of paper.

Barcode Kavita Exercise, YouTube

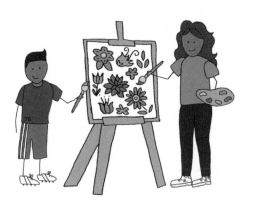

CHAPTER 8

**Be happy, not because everything is good, but
because you see the good in everything.**

—PROJECT HAPPINESS

Happiness, April 2018

AFTER SEARCHING FOR something that could give me purpose in
life, it's been so overwhelming to understand exactly what that is.
What is the purpose of life? What is the meaning? Why am I here?
Lots of people get into the same habits or follow others in being the
same way, doing the same thing and talking in a similar manner.
But each one of us is individual, and we all have our own purpose
and way of being. What's yours?

I know that I am a creative person that loves being outside in
nature, and I love painting and cooking, but the lifestyle I was leading
left me no time at all to enjoy my first loves. This part of my personality gave me happiness, and I somehow lost touch with that along
the way. But the good news is I've found it again and am indulging in
things I enjoy almost every day! I believe the purpose of life is to find
that ultimate happiness, and once you realise this, it's just amazing.
I absolutely love the days when I sketch and paint—I make them
happen much more often than ever before. I love cycling trips around

my hometown or on holiday—they give me a sense of freedom. I also love spending all that quality time with my family, especially my children. It just makes me so happy. I'm very grateful for what I have, so anything else is just a lovely surprise bonus. Most of all, I always make a point of saying thank you or adding a silly, happy emoji at the end of my messages and emails. I think it will make someone's day or at least make them smile, and if I can do that, it makes me smile too.

Another key point I realised was that I needed to keep it simple and enjoy the simple things—eating food with my family, watching a good film or even just sitting in the garden watching my puppy play. I always thought that if I had that lovely designer dress, if I could have an amazing figure or go on that cruise I always wanted, these things would make me happy. However, I've learned that material or superficial things give short-term happiness, not the one that we are all striving for. I also discovered that people might measure happiness in different ways at different stages. I am just expressing what makes me happy, and the really sad thing is that I only realised this incredible secret of happiness after nearly losing my life. Why would it take such a tragedy? A simple life is a happy life—that's my take on it.

You can really enjoy life if you are content with who you are and do the things that make you happy. Because a happy you means a happy family, and in return, a happy life! Here are five things, researched and presented by Live Science, that will help you lead a better, happier life. If you would like further information, please follow the link: *http://www.livescience.com/9824-5-happier.html*

1. Be grateful. Some study participants were asked to write letters of gratitude to people who had helped them in some way. The study found that these people reported a lasting increase in happiness—over weeks and even months—after implementing the habit. Even more surprising, sending the letter is not necessary. When people wrote letters but never delivered them to the addressee, they still reported feeling better afterwards.

2. Be optimistic. Another practice that seems to help is optimistic thinking. Study participants were asked to visualize an ideal future—for example, living with a loving and supportive partner or finding a job that was fulfilling—and describe the image in a journal entry. After doing this for a few weeks, these people too reported increased feelings of well-being.

3. Count your blessings. People who write down three good things that have happened to them every week show significant boosts in happiness, studies have found. It seems the act of focusing on the positive helps people remember reasons to be glad.

4. Use your strengths. Another study asked people to identify their greatest strengths and then try to use these strengths in new ways. For example, someone who says they have a good sense of humour could try telling jokes to lighten up business meetings or cheer up sad friends. This habit also seems to increase happiness.

5. Commit acts of kindness. It turns out helping others also helps ourselves. People who donate time or money to charity or who assist people in need report improvements in their own happiness. Sonja Lyubomirsky has created a free iPhone app called Live Happy to help people boost their well-being.

Barcode Painting

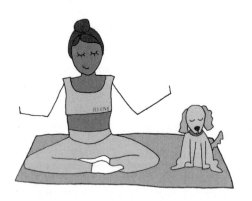

CHAPTER 9

**He who is not courageous enough to take
risks will accomplish nothing in life.**

—MUHAMMAD ALI

Try something new! May 2018
IN THE SPIRIT of trying something new, I signed up for a fitness
boot camp. I am completely dreading the thought of doing this.
This is the first time that I've tried a boot camp—I don't even know
how they work! But being the soldier I am, I'm always up for trying
something different. I sign up to go early Sunday morning whilst
the rest of my family is asleep—it was too difficult to attempt to
drag one of them along. So I'm there and doing this dynamic routine with complete strangers. Maybe it's better that I don't know
them? I inform the instructor that I am recovering from a little
thing called a brain hemorrhage that happened last year and ask
him to be mindful of how hard he is pushing me. Well, you know
what? I tried it, and it was so refreshing to exercise outside, to meet
new people—and there was great teamwork!

Although I couldn't do all the activities, the main thing is I
tried. I was so proud of myself just for getting ready in my outfit

and driving to the gym! Yes, that's a great step—well done, me. Honestly, that was the most difficult part. But the interval training—that was easy, although I was so shattered on the last round that I decided to take a bold step and do a sprint around the field instead. I came back to a 'Well done!' by the instructor. What I realised is that I can only do what I can do. I didn't need to follow anyone or keep up with anyone else, and I did something different, out of the box, and was so proud of myself that at least I tried it.

Six years prior to the SAH, I tried two new activities that have been a huge help in my recovery and are now among the loves of my life: yoga and meditation. What I don't understand is why no one told me about them when I was young. Yoga is one of the best forms of exercise, with a mix of stretching, keeping active and breathing techniques. The benefits I've received over the years have been so great for mind, body and soul. I have now been practising yoga for nine years.

I went back to the Zumba classes that I used to love. Joining in with a group of dancers to some Latin or Spanish music is really uplifting, but unknown to me, a side effect I have now is that my co-ordination is not the same as it used to be. I went to the class a year after the SAH and couldn't follow the instructions in time, waved my right arm instead of my left and started to bump into others! I was so embarrassed. At the time I thought I was out of my routine and just needed to get back into it. But later I learned that after a brain injury, many people have co-ordination issues. This can be from cognitive issues as the brain is instructing the body to move, and the response may be slightly scrambled on the way. So I'm just a little out of sync now. If I didn't try new activities to keep up my exercise, I wouldn't have found what I love doing now: meditation, yoga, walking. I tried different types of exercise to see what worked for me, and yoga makes me smile each time I practise.

Life is full of opportunities, and sometimes we get worried that if we try something new, we may fail. The key is to think, 'I will try this, and if it's not good for me, then it's okay'. If you want to try a new activity, don't be scared to make that bold step. Making the decision to go is the most difficult bit. If no one wants to accompany you, then just go by yourself! You are the one who wants to do this, so enjoy it—you might meet some new friends. Don't try to keep up or follow everyone else. This is your life, and if you want to think outside the box and do something different, then you should. Being confident enough to try something new is brave. It opens your life up to possibilities, and it could change your life path and inspire your imagination!

6 reasons why you should try something new:

1. Because you don't want to live with regrets.

2. Because you never know what you might find.

3. Because it will give you self-confidence.

4. Because you'll be more interesting.

5. Because YOLO.

6. Because no one ever accomplished anything by letting their fear conquer them.

Barcode Dancing Again, YouTube

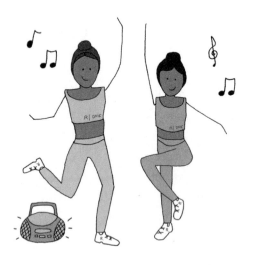

CHAPTER 10

**You never know how strong you are until
being strong is the only choice you have.**

—Bob Marley

Bee Courageous, August 2018

How to be courageous in life? This is a difficult one. I think everyone has different levels of experience that would determine their courage. But what a great quote we have here from Bob Marley! It's especially close to my heart, being a fellow Leo and having just celebrated my forty-second birthday. It made me think about some of the many challenges throughout my life that have shaped my courage. I would like to share these with you, as I believe each one has had an effect on me and how I've dealt with situations as I've grown. They have definitely made me stronger—someone once said to me, 'The difficult experiences you have shape who you are!'

Here are my highlights and how they have impacted my courage:

- Living without my parents at a very young age. I learned to fend for myself during those years in India as a child. My sister and I lived with our grandparents and uncle and aunt for a few years because my parents were starting a new business venture and also wanted us to understand our culture and where we came from.

- Migraines. I used to suffer from these as a child; stress or exhaustion triggered them. I learned to stay calm and focus on only doing what I could at the time.

- Catching malaria on a work trip. This is still with me. I don't really think about it; I just live with what I have. It's just another thing I have to deal with.

- Crohn's disease. In my early twenties, I was diagnosed and put on mounds of medication. I have changed my diet and am now medication-free! I gave up eating meat—Crohn's has made me eat healthier!

- Arthritis. A side effect from Crohn's, this is in most of my joints. It takes over when I'm cold or tired. I try and keep a source of warmth nearby.

- My father's passing. This also happened in my early twenties. It has taught me to not take life for granted because it is too short.

- Losing a pregnancy. This happened twice, once at a very early stage. The second was a very difficult situation; it was ectopic, so as well as losing my future child, I had my fallopian tube removed. This scarred me physically and emotionally. It made me realise I should just appreciate the two wonderful children I already have.

- Subarachnoid brain hemorrhage. This near-death experience had the greatest impact. Four operations later, with a shunt inserted in my brain, which is now implanted for life, I still ploughed my way through this huge event which I don't think I will ever understand fully as to why it happened to me and the implications of the aftereffects. Maybe I will never have closure on this?

- Meningitis. I caught this during my time in hospital. This infection can cause severe damage but staying positive helped me through it.

- Hair loss. This was a side effect of the brain hemorrhage trauma I experienced. I learned to see that my appearance was just the wrapping and the person inside was what really mattered. It grew back!

- High anxiety. My mental health is controlled with regular therapy sessions and neuropsychology. These have helped me and my family in so many ways. I am now a happier me!

Let's think about the experiences that have made us courageous and stay positive in dealing with new situations. I am doing a speaking event in Philadelphia this September for The Bee Foundation, whose motto is 'Bee Aware, Bee Courageous and Bee Happy'. It is an amazing charity.

The mission of The Bee Foundation is to raise awareness of brain aneurysms and increase funding for innovative research that changes lives. We are building a robust and dynamic brain aneurysm research community with our Scientific Advisory Board, donors and network of researchers interested in grant funding to support meaningful research. Our community, anchored by our grant recipients, is committed to advancing brain aneurysm research. I feel honoured to share my experiences to be able to help others. For more information on the Honey Bash Ball, please follow the link below: *https://www.thebeefoundation.org/meet-honey-bash-guest-speaker-kavita-basi/* BEE COURAGEOUS!

Courage has to come from within, and you need to be brave to move forward.

According to the Cambridge Dictionary online, the meaning of courage is '*the ability to control your fear in a dangerous or difficult situation*'.

Barcode Kavi, Soho farmhouse milestone

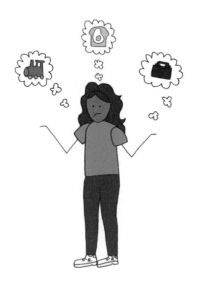

CHAPTER 11

**If you don't like how things are,
change it! You're not a tree.**

—JIM ROHN

Anxiety, June 2018

WHAT IS ANXIETY? There are so many different levels, and some can be so severe they could lead to a panic attack. (If you haven't experienced one, it can be so overwhelming it almost feels like a heart attack.) I want to share one of my personal anxiety stories and also help you with tools that may alleviate this condition.

It was during our Spanish Adventure, August 2017. We used to go on lots of adventures with the family before my illness, and they almost became a must for every school break and even some weekends in between. We were constantly preoccupied with planning the next trip. It was quite stressful—not to mention expensive! Going through a life-changing event like an SAH will shift your priorities. We don't plan like we used to, and we stay home on most breaks now, so when we do go away, it's much more appreciated—a new, exciting adventure. Now it feels like I'm doing a lot of things for the first time, even though I have travelled all over the world with my job for over twenty years, experiencing so much culture and life. But now it's so different. I am looking at the world through a new pair of eyes, and it is amazing!

I had a form of anxiety attack one morning while travelling by train between two cities in Spain because I had more than four things to do (you might think that's nothing, but to me it's an overload). This was affecting me; I could feel the build-up inside my head, the stress levels increasing. It was just too much.

- Check out of the hotel.

- Eat breakfast.

- Send the suitcases down with concierge.

- Check the children's cases are packed.

- Find out the distance to the train station from the hotel.

- Check out (yes, it was going through my mind again!).

What others fail to understand is that when I have a timed situation and lots to do, stress can start to build up inside, and then my coping mechanism is to fly away! I used to be the one who was calm and collected and kept everything together. I looked to my husband, and even though he knows most of what I'm going through, he doesn't seem to connect with the fact that sometimes it's all too much for me and I just need him to take control. Any effort will help me. Thankfully, after telling my family about how I was feeling, we had breakfast, the children were ready and packed, and Deepak got us to the train station.

To understand more about anxiety, follow this link: *https://www. anxietyuk.org.uk/anxiety-type/generalised-anxiety-disorder/?gclid=C-jwKCAjw5uTMBRAYEiwA5HxQNhtUNhJPa2BkLmSr8o23Ts8B_DQbeWJozRwOsK8CalKg485oKtoi3BoCQ5UQAvD_BwE*

5 things to do when anxiety is building up:

1. Get comfortable. The first step in overcoming anxiety is to recognize that your job is to make yourself as comfortable as possible until the feeling passes. And it will pass. While you are waiting for the anxiety to pass, remind yourself that this feeling will go away and concentrate on making yourself comfortable physically and emotionally. To increase physical comfort, find a comfortable position, stretch your muscles and loosen any tight clothing you are wearing. To increase emotional comfort, continue with the following methods.

2. Use calming self-talk. Much of what we say to ourselves when experiencing anxiety causes us to feel more anxious. Tell yourself calming phrases such as 'This feeling will pass', 'I will get through this', 'I am safe right now', 'I am feeling anxious now, but soon I will be calm', 'I can feel my heart rate gradually slowing down'.

3. Acknowledge and accept the anxiety. Fighting the anxiety makes it stronger. Paradoxically, accepting that you are feeling anxious can cause the anxiety to go away. If you are feeling brave enough to try the following, it is one of the most powerful anxiety treatment strategies: For ten minutes, try to make yourself as anxious as possible. Think anxious thoughts. Try to get your anxiety to increase to the highest imaginable level. When your anxiety reaches a 10 out of 10, good! Now try to keep it there for at least five minutes. You will probably find that you are not able to keep your anxiety at a high level. This is a type of exposure technique in which you face your fears—and they vanish.

4. Distract yourself. Distraction is an effective way of putting your mind on something other than the anxiety symptoms you are experiencing. It is difficult for the mind to focus on more than one thing at once. If you find something to focus on intently, your mind will not be able to maintain the anxiety for long.

5. Relax. Relaxation is the body's natural anxiety cure because it reverses the stress response. Use quick relaxation techniques to induce this response. This will counter the body's stress response and reduce anxiety symptoms. Click below to learn more about how to quickly achieve the relaxation response.

http://www.innerhealthstudio.com/overcoming-anxiety.html

Barcode Anxiety YouTube

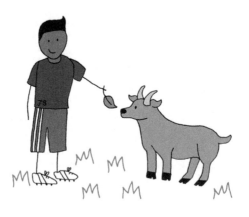

CHAPTER 12

**If happiness is the goal—and it should be—
then adventures should be a priority.**

—Richard Branson

Every day can be an adventure! September 2018
This chapter is inspired by the movie Goodbye Christopher
Robin. Every day seems to be an adventure, and I try my best to
live in the moment.

Our Greek Adventure, in August 2018, was such a wonderful
experience. My children were nearly adults, so the holiday was more
like enjoying time with my friends. *Athens—home of Athena, goddess
of war and wisdom*—is surrounded by ancient Greek structures,
including the Acropolis, and what an amazing sight it is! We trek
right up to the top and explore this magnificent ruin. I am overwhelmed by the sheer size of the structures and the massive effort,
in those days, of bringing the building materials up there to be
constructed to make this momentous World Heritage site.

Even though we visit *the Parthenon—Athena's temple*—in
the evening, around five o'clock, the sun is still scorching, but
this doesn't stop the vast number of visitors at the top of the hill

exploring the Acropolis. I sit on the rocks at the side with my husband and just look around, absorbing this wonderful moment and watching my children in awe of the surroundings. We can see the whole city from here—the white buildings are glistening in the sun, and it is truly magical. I want to know more about this place, learn why it was built and what the representations of these overbearing structures were. I look at my thirteen-year-old son, who has to complete a school project this summer, and cheekily ask, 'Should we do your project about Greece?' This is how I am going to add to my learning as well as spend quality time with my child.

Later, we walk through the cobbled city streets, passing some old musicians playing traditional Greek tunes. It feels so natural and cultural. We enter a very quiet street, and I start to panic that we're going to be lost in some derelict place, but in the distance, I see some fairy lights and a few steps leading up to a beautiful traditional taverna filled with colourful flowers and mounds of greenery. The owner greets us and tells us that the hotel has booked us the best table in the house, a rooftop space overlooking the whole city. At this point the sun is setting, and the city lights are starting to appear. I can't contain my excitement and just want my family to take in the same happiness I'm feeling.

We are staying in a beautiful boutique hotel called The Margi, which is located further south on the tip of the Greek coast, approximately thirty minutes away from Athens. We are cared for here by very attentive staff with a warm, welcoming nature. It's a small hotel with a grand charm about it. The rooms are cosy but modern, and we have a lovely balcony overlooking the pool area and parts of the city. As soon as we walk in, the aroma of fresh flowers and richly scented perfumed candles fills the reception area. I talk to the waiter in the morning—his name is Andreas—learning new words that I can say in Greek, like 'fharristoe' (thank you) and 'para colla' (you're welcome) and 'calai meera' (good morning). Excuse my spelling—I've written these how I heard them.

Whenever I travel, I always feel the need to understand the culture and immerse myself in it. So to be polite and learn a little— why not? The other member of the team I became very friendly with was Aphrodite, who helped to make my experience so enjoyable by booking us a short tour of a local farm. The hotel produce was all organic from farm to table, and yes, they owned their own farm! I was so ecstatic about this. However, the tours were very expensive and took too long, as we only had a couple of days in Athens, so I kindly asked Aphrodite if my family could just do a short visit to see it.

She made it possible, and we had the best time feeding the goats—especially Stelios, a giant white goat larger than me! He had tufted hair on top and a tufted chin—my son said he looked like Elvis Presley—huge, curled-up horns and brilliant white fur. I had never seen anything so magnificent. We then did some grape-picking, learned about the fruit and vegetables and how they were grown and even met Billie, a rescued donkey that had been maltreated and overworked. He was now in this sanctuary, having the time of his life. As we were leaving, the farm keeper, Meehra, kindly gave me a brown package filled with grapes and chillies to take back with me. It was just the best time, and I loved each moment. Being on this farm was our little adventure, being in Athens was our adventure. It felt so magical as each experience seemed to feel like a new treasure that gave us a glimmer of happiness, even in the simplest of things.

We were then off to Khalkidhiki, where we would meet my sister and her family to continue our Greek Adventure. Since my SAH I have had this force behind me pushing me to learn more and experience new things. This happens each day, each moment. It's as if I've gone back to being a child, one that can absorb more information than my adult self. It is very intriguing, though, and the more I'm learning, the happier I am. It could be that I feel I don't have much time left or that the impact to my head has aligned my brain in some way to take in more information. Whatever the reason, I am enjoying this journey. So watching the Christopher Robin movie reminded me of how, through a child's perspective, a simple journey that may seem very normal and basic can be an amazing discovery that unfolds to tell a beautiful story. I try to share my experiences in this way; since my illness, each one feels like the first ever discovery, and I'm back to being a child like Christopher Robin.

Barcode Acropolis

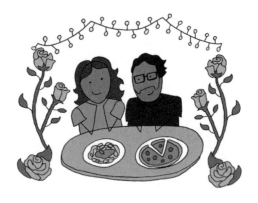

CHAPTER 13

You are the universe, you aren't in the universe.

—Eckhart Tolle

Hidden Gems, October 2018

It's very easy to get into a habit of following others and doing the normal things when taking a trip—going to the top ten 'where to be seen' restaurants where you know the menu inside out or staying in the same recommended hotels. Yes, it becomes a little repetitive, so you really know how your day is going to go. *But* have you ever moved out of your comfort zone to explore and go with the flow, as if you are leaving it all to the Universe?

We took a trip to USA when I was invited as the guest of honour and a keynote speaker for a very worthy charity, The Bee Foundation for Aneurysm Awareness, at their Honey Bash Ball in Philadelphia. We thought it would be a great idea to add a couple more days to the trip so my husband and I could have a short romantic break together in New York and Philadelphia.

I must have been to New York over fifteen times, for work and pleasure, in my twenty-four years of work. Each time we stayed either near Fifth Avenue's main shopping area or on the doorstep of Central

Park. This time I decided to book us into a small boutique hotel called *Hotel Hugo* in downtown Soho, a quirky, hip area I have always loved.

My husband likes his comforts and was worried. 'I'm not sure about gong here—how do you know if it's good? We will be really far out.' I, on the other hand, had done my research. It had great reviews and a rooftop bar, which was one of the top hot spots for budding professionals to hang out after work. The interior design, with shiny mahogany finish almost everywhere, gave it a seventies retro feel. Each room was small but cosy, with all linen marked *HH*, giving it an almost celebrity personalisation. The restaurant was Italian, so it ticked all the boxes!

As we entered, I was pleasantly surprised by the very lovely, floor-to-ceiling green wall features behind reception and in the main dining area. These walls were full of plants that were trimmed and pruned on a regular basis to look perfect. And of course, the very helpful staff made us feel cosy and at home instantly.

It was late, and we ate at the hotel. The waiter recommended a fabulous meal for us. I had pasta with eggplant baked and served in a cast iron dish. Deepak ate something called chicken on a brick—a piece of tender, roasted chicken placed neatly on a bed of quinoa salsa. In the middle of the table, we had a yummy, tangy kale salad with hints of orange segments highlighting a fresh summer taste. We then went to explore the rooftop *Bar Hugo*. It had such a cool Mexican vibe, with comfy sofa seating, small, colourful tables and fairy lights above creating a magical ceiling. However, we were just a little too tired to appreciate it, and we had an early start the next day.

We were both working the following day. We both work as consultants in the fashion industry, connecting brands with suppliers and vice versa but also planning to have our own ethical fashion brands one day. But before we headed to the office, it was time for a much-loved breakfast. I had visited this beautiful French brasserie, *Lafayette Grand Café,* a while before for a quick healthy snack takeaway, so I wanted to visit again and let my dear husband enjoy some great food. I met the owner this time, who said she had been on a yoga retreat and loved to connect with like-minded people. It was meant to be that we were there at that point, eating in that café, talking to this lovely woman. Her ethos was exactly how I see mine, and my own ethical yoga clothing brand would just be amazing.

Deepak and I finished work, and again I did not want to do the normal New York shopping experience. So we both decided to pay our respects at Ground Zero and the World Trade Center. The experience of this was something else. Seeing the vast, empty space and the names of all those lost was truly overwhelming. We walked back to the hotel, looking at the quirky shops and cafés along the way. It was so great to be able to just live life in the moment and be spontaneous. To experience things in our own time, without being pressured into a routine or watching the clock, is something else.

After a rest, we asked the hotel staff if there was a local Italian restaurant nearby (yes, it is our favourite cuisine!). They directed us to a quaint, small place in the middle of Soho, walking distance. We entered a little Italian escape, *Palma,* off Cornelia Street, with an indoor garden filled with plants, roses and fairy lights—beautiful surroundings. It was as if we were in the heart of a family home, with candlelit steps up the side to a balcony overlooking the courtyard. The staff were so lovely and accommodated our dietary requirements. It didn't feel like we were in the bustling city of New York. We had been transported to another place, and I loved every minute there.

Philadelphia was another adventure. We took the train from Penn Station, opposite Madison Square Garden. I sat down and instantly started talking to a young woman sitting opposite who was a part-time actor, and we talked about our favourite program, *Grand Designs!* We also talked about how *Harry Potter* books have changed lives and how life was such a surprise, and then our journey was suddenly over! It was so helpful to connect with someone and enjoy a conversation. Mr Basi, on the other hand, slept all the way! Driving to the hotel through the city of Philadelphia felt very stately, and there was a grandeur about the place, but I needed to sleep before my big appearance at the charity ball and wanted to save all my energy after this.

I was proud to be the guest of honour, seated at the first table. I spoke in front of 160 people, including many medical professionals, patients, families and carers. I was so proud of myself—it felt good to, hopefully, make a difference by being there and sharing my experiences. The full speech is available on The Bee Foundation's Facebook page if you wish to read it.

The following day, I was up at five, ready and excited to explore Philadelphia! As we walked through the heart of the city, the buildings reminded me of Washington, DC. Compared to the skyscrapers of modern New York, Philadelphia showed a lot of history, and I was pleasantly surprised by its colonial ambiance. We stopped at a brunch café called *Chez Ben* attached to a *Renaissance* hotel on Chestnut Street, in the old city. It was a lovely place for breakfast and had a café counter with quality coffees, fresh juices and buttery pastries.

Another famous, not-so-hidden gem from this prestigious city had to be the *Franklin Institute Science Museum*, where we learned about the famous author, printer, political theorist, politician, Freemason, postmaster, scientist, inventor, humourist, civic activist, statesman and diplomat. He was a legend! Now, we didn't have time to do both the museum and the institute, so we visited the institute. My highlight here had to be sitting in the huge, 360-degree video dome watching the BBC's *Blue Planet II*! It felt as if I was at sea and could touch what was in front of me. I did not want to miss a thing. Mr Basi, on the other hand, got comfortable in his seat and fell asleep again!

Back on the street, we could hear loud music and cheering. The Puerto Rican Day Parade was passing by! We joined it and walked alongside, clapping and cheering. The music, cars, motorbikes and costumes were so cultural and exciting to watch. Mr Basi is an avid *Rocky* fan, and as we were walking to the end of the parade route, his eyes lit up when he saw the famous *Rocky statue and steps*. We ran up them as if we were in the film and recorded it on video. When we reached the top, we took in the amazing view—it was as if we had both been transported back to age fourteen, getting giddy over such a simple thing. We had an evening flight, but before heading back, we ate at a French bistro called *Pietro's* on Walnut Street. This neighbourhood was very cool and chic, full of trendy stores and cafés. The four days we had felt like a two-week indulgence of amazing adventure. The hidden gems made it all so worthwhile. Try to live in the moment—you never know where it might take you.

5 things to help you live in the moment:

1. Wake up in the morning and don't look at your phone.

2. Delete all prearranged plans for the day and go somewhere that gives you a happy vibe.

3. Go for a walk, either locally or to a beautiful park (make sure it's safe), and look at what surrounds you. Say hello and smile at everyone you see.

4. Go to a local café. Invite a friend or go on your own with a notebook—you might just enjoy jotting down some happy thoughts.

5. Eat something you've never tried before. It's an adventure, remember, so just go for it!

Barcode Rocky steps

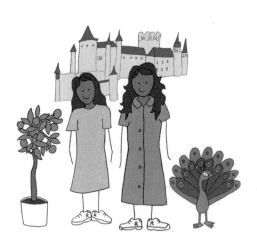

CHAPTER 14

**We live in a wonderful world that is full
of beauty, charm and adventure. There is
no end to the adventures we can have if
only we seek them with our eyes open.**

—JAWAHARLAL NEHRU

Sevilla, one of the most beautiful places, April 2019
WHEN SOMEONE SUGGESTED Seville as a holiday destination to me,
I really did not know what to expect. If you haven't yet visited,
then you are missing one of the most beautiful cities on Earth.
Imagine stepping outside into streets filled with orange and lemon
trees, with the acoustics of Spanish guitar echoing through sunlit
historical buildings, and being greeted by colourful peacocks in the
gardens of the Real Alcázar Palace. This is Sevilla.

*Seville (in Spanish, Sevilla) is a big city in the south of Spain, in
Europe. A large river called Guadalquivir runs through it, the only great
navigable river in Spain. Currently, it runs from the Gulf of Cádiz to
Seville, but in Roman times, it was navigable to Córdoba. The city of Seville
is the capital of the Spanish region called Andalusia.* I simply had to write
about this wonderful place and share the amazing sights, streets and

cafés I visited during my stay. I can only share a small selection of the images; however, if you follow my Instagram (@kavita_basi), you will be able to see much more of this mesmerizing place. Now, this was my second time visiting here; I was accompanying my daughter, who was studying at a Spanish school for a week. I took the opportunity to get some rest, sunshine and some great inspiration.

It didn't disappoint. We had stayed at the great Hotel Alfonso XIII on our previous visit two years earlier, but I wanted to experience more of the culture this time by staying in the heart of the city, at the Hotel Corral del Ray (*https://www.corraldelrey.com/corral-del-rey*). It was March, a great time to visit as it was just starting to get warm. The taxi driver dropped us a little way down from the narrow, cobbled street and directed us to walk with our luggage toward the street corner, where we would find a large glass door lined with intricately designed iron bars set in a rectangular stone archway. I was already feeling like this place was going to be my second home for the next week. I had taken a week off work for myself, even though I was accompanying Jasmine for her work experience and intensive Spanish education. I needed some time for myself, to clear my mind, be inspired and (relax because work had been so overwhelming with the many challenges of the fashion industry. I needed some time to think about what I wanted to do. After being through such a life-changing experience, I felt I should just focus on what could make me happy. This trip was going to be that sanctuary and the turning point of my new career.

The hotel comprised of three buildings, the main reception area and two villas opposite. We would have our own entrance hall, library and chill-out area.

Here is some info from the website: '*The Corral Del Ray is located in the old quarter of Barrio Alfalfa, Sevilla just five minutes from the Cathedral, the original 17th century casa Palacio has been meticulously restored and converted into a small private luxury boutique hotel.*' The team at the hotel were very attentive. The small group of women were so friendly and helpful, making our stay even more comfortable and definitely an experience to remember.

My days started with navigating my way through the historic cobbled streets and stopping at every corner for a photo opportunity—yes, *every* corner. As we walked through the old town on our first day, there was a commotion going on near the Plaza Nueva. A parade was entering the square from Plaza San Francisco, and a competition between various South American regions was taking place! Watching this huge cultural display was so exciting and definitely one of the highlights of the trip.

We celebrated Jasmine's nineteenth birthday at a favourite restaurant of ours built within the ancient Arab baths—San Marco, an Italian eatery visited by many celebrities, including Madonna! The food was exquisite, and we were serenaded by a local band playing their instruments live during our meal. It was perfect—the anniversary of the date I went into the hospital that frightening night suffering a brain hemorrhage. This meal, combined with Jasmine's birthday, was going to create special new memories.

There is a huge Arabic influence in Sevilla due to the invasion many years back and the proximity of the regions. It is quite apparent in most of the architecture around the city, which is classified as Mudejar, a blend of Moorish, Arabian and Gothic influences. Some of the structures include the Catedral de Sevilla, Casa de Pilatos and the Real Alcázar Palace.

If you are a *Game of Thrones* fan, you will be pleased to know that Seville was one of the main locations for this hugely popular series. You will recognise the scenes that took place in the Real Alcázar Palace and in the Parque de Maria Luisa. This place is a film director's dream due to the amazing landscape and, of course, the weather! The Plaza de España was host to a great film—*Star Wars Episode II: Attack of the Clones*. Parque de Maria Luisa was formerly the gardens of the palace of San Telmo and was donated to the city by the Duchess of Montpensier. Its archaeology museum hosts many interesting artefacts.

Now, I like to eat early, between six thirty and seven thirty, if possible. If you are like me, then you will have to have tapas as an early evening snack, as the restaurants do not open till eight thirty for dinner! One of my reigning favourite tapas places is Bar Catedral Sevilla on the bustling street of Calle Mateos Gago, where you can watch magnificent horse-drawn carriages go by.

We completed our cultural stay by enrolling in a dancing class at the famous Museo de Flamenco. This felt like I was taking in the whole Spanish experience in its full entirety. I rediscovered my love for art, rebalanced my chakras and also made some very important decisions for my life ahead. This was a memorable time for me, and one I would never forget. If you have followed my story from my first book, *Room 23*, then you will understand my passion of having my own lifestyle company. It was born here in Seville—Jardin Living. I hope you will see more of this over the next few years. What a trip! Cristina, Isabel, Carmen and Chaima at the Corral del Rey, thank you for making our stay so memorable.

Wish list guide for Sevilla:

- Visit and attend Mass at Seville Cathedral.
- Climb to the top of La Giralda, the bell tower at the cathedral.
- Row a boat in Plaza de España.
- Ride bikes around Parque de Maria Luisa.
- Visit the Seville Archaeology Museum.
- Visit some of the many art galleries.
- Ride in a horse-drawn carriage through Santa Cruz in the old town.
- Eat at Petit Comité, a quaint dinner place near the river.

- Eat at San Marco, a restaurant built in the ancient Arab baths.
- Take a flamenco-dancing class!

Barcode Sevilla

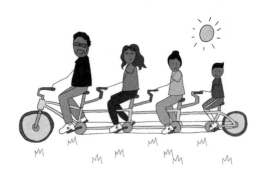

CHAPTER 15

Either you run the day or the day runs you.

—JIM ROHN

Positive Affirmations, June 2019

TODAY IS GOING to be a good day☺. Do you wake up in the morning thinking 'I really can't be bothered' or 'I am so tired and I would like to just go back to sleep'? News! You are not the only one—this is quite normal! We all have sluggish mornings when we just want to wake up and do nothing, some more often than others because we are all different and have varied energy levels. Sometimes we just want to have a duvet day. Ooooh, I love a duvet day!

This is even more apparent if you have been through a serious, life-threatening illness, like me. Fatigue and mental health are a huge part of my side effects, and what keeps me going is the fact that I am here, I'm alive and I will be okay! Waking up in the morning with a positive attitude can completely change my day. Thinking positively before going to sleep can really affect the quality of your sleep and completely change your mood when you wake up the next day. It is a fact because I'm actually doing it. Now each morning I feel energised, happy, positive and ready to take on the challenges of the day. It feels *amazing*!

I am sharing five affirmations you can repeat to yourself each day. I like to wake up feeling that I want to make a difference to other people, make them positive and happy—this is my goal—but I also like to keep myself in check. A happy you means a happy family, which is really important to remember because your vibe attracts your tribe!

When I was younger and living in India, I loved being outdoors, cycling around the neighbourhood with my friends. It was something I could do that gave me a little freedom, and—especially in warm weather—it was lovely to feel the breeze against my skin. On my recent trips with my family, where possible, I make a point of hiring bikes. Even though I can't do a long trek, I enjoy a little stroll, especially when we go somewhere warm.

One time in particular, we visited a beautiful city called Lucca in Italy, thirty minutes away from Pisa. The city is very quaint—it's enclosed by ancient walls, and when you enter, there is only one way in, through an arch in the wall. Lucca is full of little cobbled streets and local businesses selling shoes, clothes, fruit, baskets and more. It embraces everything local, which gives it a strong feeling of community. On the day we arrived, we had a quiet meal nearby and walked back to the hotel.

The next morning, after breakfast, I packed my sketchbook and pencils, and off we went to explore with the children on our bikes. We went to the edge of the city walls and climbed a few short steps. As we reached the top, it was so amazing to see that the rooftops of the walls had been made into a wide path with greenery alongside—a social space, a circular park for walking and cycling that surrounded the city. People were walking with their dogs, eating ice cream or jogging with friends, and other families were cycling too. We could see the whole city from up there, and it was breath-taking. It was such an amazing feeling to cycle on this beautiful pathway with such amazing views! More recently, on a trip to Croatia, we took out bikes for an afternoon, riding along the coastline of the island of Brac.

My cycling has continued at home since my husband bought me a pink bike with a basket! So I have found enjoyment in cycling again. It's a positive change that I have put back into my life. Below are some other key changes to get you to a positive, happy life. I promise, making these changes will keep you positive and happy. They will change your life.

If you are surrounded by negative people, remove yourself and try and change your circle. Look after your thinking. If you don't like the food you are eating, make a meal plan and change your weekly meals. Look after your body. If you feel uneasy about your work or job, then take the plunge and change it! Yes, I know it's easier said than done, but take baby steps, do one thing at a time. Look after your happiness.

5 daily reminders:

1. I am amazing.
2. I can do anything.
3. Positivity is a choice.
4. I celebrate my individuality.
5. I am prepared to succeed.

Barcode Positive vibes, Croatia cycling

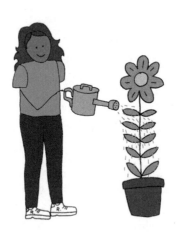

CHAPTER 16

If you can dream it, you can do it.

—Walt Disney

Sustainable Living, April 2020

THE WORD 'SUSTAINABLE' is such a broad term. Everyone is talking about it, but I have been throwing out these comments for years. You can ask my children☺. I interpret it as trying to do things in a better way that will help our environment and future generations. I am trying new ways to lead a more eco-friendly lifestyle, and it's actually quite liberating! Unfortunately, though, we are surrounded by so many non-sustainable things that we are all inclined to buy because they are either more convenient or cheaper than the sustainable alternative. Does that sound about right?

I started thinking about this seven years ago at work. I became very interested in social change and behaviour, especially in the younger generations—seeing the way my children thought, how they received their media and what content was shown. It was so interesting and actually made sense. The information they were receiving was showing that they needed to be more empathetic towards people and kinder to our environment because ecosystems were diminishing. This generation was growing and was to be our next generation—their exposure to media had started to create this want towards protecting our environment, their future environment. I wanted to help them, I wanted to make a difference, and the only way I knew how was from my past experience and how I could use this in creating better ways of using our ecosystems—did you know the fashion industry is the second-largest polluter in the world? This made me feel very sad, so I wanted to do something that would change the way people bought into apparel. But that is another story that you will, hopefully, read in my next book!

To fast forward to present day, I am now changing habits in my home so we can actively live in a cleaner, better way that will not only help our environment but encourage others to do the same. I buy products for my home that are ethically made, have fewer additives, do less harm to our planet, use eco-friendly dyes and, most of all, have a lovely, great big graphic on the front that says **'vegan'** or **'eco'**—ha ha!

My journey towards sustainable living has been part of my life for a long time. I wanted to become an architect at a very young age and studied architecture in my A levels. I loved the notion of producing buildings or interiors using recycled or organic materials. So now I am channelling this positive thinking into all other areas of my lifestyle. It began with food and drink—changing the products I bought, checking the packages and becoming a pescatarian at the age of twenty-eight. At present I have more days where I'm vegetarian or vegan.

My cleaning products, even stationery and home furnishings, including paper products for kitchen and bath, are chosen after a lot of research. Yes, it is a little time-consuming and expensive in the beginning, but once I got the products that suited my home, it was an absolute breeze thereafter. So, my goal is not only for me to change but to share these ideas with others so they can also make informed choices.

If you want to learn more about sustainable living, please go to my YouTube channel or IGTV channel, where I share the products I buy for my lifestyle. You can also search *#BetterLiving* and *#JardinLiving*. COVID-19 is affecting people in so many ways—buying only what's necessary due to lack of income or realising the need for less when there are fewer activities to explore. The experience of COVID has really changed mindsets, so let's all try and do our part to change what we can for a better, cleaner future.

YouTube: *https://www.youtube.com/watch?v=NT3lR9ss36E*

IGTV: *https://www.instagram.com/tv/B-q9_4Fnvys/*

Barcode Sustainable living #Kavitalks

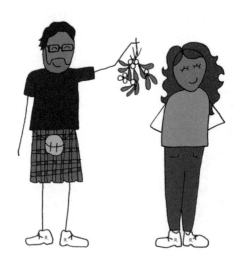

CHAPTER 17

Everything in the Universe is within you. Ask all from yourself.

—RUMI

It's Christmas, but I'm tired! December 2018

I LOVE CHRISTMAS, and I love the joy it brings; however, it became such a challenging time of year for me as a mum after suffering my SAH. High anxiety, claustrophobia, difficulty in multitasking, extreme fatigue, indecisiveness and short-term memory loss are just a few of the side effects! I know these are normal traits of stroke survivors, but after being a high-powered VP in a global fashion company, it really knocked my confidence.

Just the thought of going shopping in a crowded environment or choosing a suitable gift among too many options or being in the hustle and bustle of the Christmas markets frightens me—someone might knock my head! Of course, then I have to multitask and wrap the gifts with tags and names (I forget names constantly), which is especially difficult when you are part of a big network of family and friends—there are so many presents!

Because I am a *survivor*, I have created tools to adapt to my situation: spreadsheets, lists on my phone for the gifts that I need to get. I like to shop on the internet to get them bought, wrapped and delivered to the right recipient—so much easier! I have also started to send out a digital card to all my contacts rather than trying to remember names and posting them. Also, this helps to preserve the environment, so I'm saving trees! I prefer to go to a smaller, local Christmas market rather than the big city ones so I can have a sense of space and comfort.

Yes, it has all changed for me, but I'm extremely lucky that I have a very supportive family around me that understand what I'm going through. Sometimes you just need a rest. My husband has switched roles with me and now takes on the challenges of being the multitasking parent! Actually he is father and mother. It's quite endearing to observe.

If you find yourself struggling during the holiday season, adapt to what you can or just ask someone to help you☺. My first book, *Room 23*, chronicles some of my experiences, which I have shared to help others. You can buy at Amazon or go to the header on my website for links to purchase from other stores.

December 2019

I was dreading the whole process of getting ready for Christmas. so we decided to meet my family in Scotland. Jasmine was studying there, and it would be an opportunity to see the city. Plus, we wouldn't have to do all the dinner preparations, cook, clean and get the house ready—it would all be done for us! The only thing I had to do was get the presents ready. It was a new way for me to cope with my anxiety and fatigue at Christmas.

Barcode – Xmas, December 2019, Scotsman

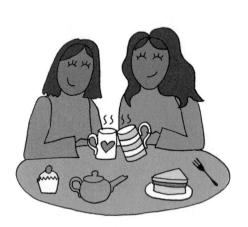

CHAPTER 18

Your vibe attracts your tribe.

—Anonymous

Surround yourself with positivity and food!

A very close friend of mine before my hemorrhage got in touch with me recently, and it was lovely to see that familiar face and talk about what we used to do together. However, it wasn't the same, and even though remembering those magical happy moments made me smile for a minute, I was no longer in the same situation. I tried to explain that this new me had to be embraced—it was not just part of who I am, but the whole new me—in the same way, and being part of my life now was more important than ever. Why hadn't this friend been around for me? What I didn't realise was that they had their own situation, their own troubles, and the timing clashed with my needs. I may think my needs are more significant, so does everyone think theirs are more important in their own way?

So this is one way of looking at it. The other side of my thought process is this. Say there is a monumental change in your life that affects your whole family in so many ways, and you are at your lowest point, where you need support and help, but your closest friends are not around. When you have been through the difficult times and picked yourself up and are now thriving in your personal and professional life, and these friends reappear, is this friendship? I think everyone has to work out their own assumptions and values and see what is good for them and what isn't. Surround yourself with the right people, the ones who lift your spirits and keep you happy as well as celebrating your highs and supporting you during your lows.

Also, on another point, I'm a very obsessive person, becoming more so with time. Whether it's age or the illness, it doesn't matter—what matters is it makes me want something so much that I will do anything, like a dog with a bone. Not in a bad way, but in a determined way. Now, this is great when I'm in a professional role, as I get the job done, but it doesn't entirely work in a family situation, like getting your teenage son out of bed at six thirty in the morning to take the dog for a walk. Yes, six thirty in the morning on Sunday! I can now understand why he goes bonkers on me. I'm a dog with a bone! He is my family, and hopefully, he will understand. I try and explain as much as possible about my illness and why I get this way. I'm also obsessed with food, experiences, my family, Brandi—all in all, with life!

I have a small group of very close friends that I like to go for walks or have brunch or afternoon tea with and discuss the joys of family life and just have a laugh. This, to me, is true friendship, and there are no expectations. To genuinely be happy for someone with a true heart and love them as they are is the only way to enjoy friendship and life. Since I have removed the negativity of certain people and situations, my life has definitely become happier. I'm enjoying who I'm with, and everything doesn't need to be a comparison, a race to be better or look better.

Just be yourself, and the rest with follow. This is something you realise as you get older. Why was this secret kept from younger me twenty years ago, when I was starting out? What I have learned and adapted to is that it doesn't matter—at least I know it now.

Barcode, Food with friends

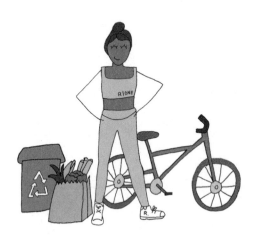

CHAPTER 19

**Cherish the natural world, because you're
a part of it and you depend on it.**

—Sir David Attenborough

For most of my childhood and adult life, I have been surrounded by the fashion industry, starting with my parents' little store in Durham, a small, beautiful city in the northeast of England. It was a compact shop, but it seemed to have everything! We had the latest trends from various wholesalers around the UK in women's, men's and children's clothing, and in the corner, we had a uniform section for all the surrounding schools, plus other areas containing underwear, socks, tights, hats and more. My siblings and I would spend weekends and holidays helping out, as that was what we needed to do to support our parents in those days. It was hard work, but fun. Unpacking the boxes was the best—we couldn't wait to find out if there was something we liked and if our father would let us take it home! We also enjoyed the staff parties, which were the best as we watched everyone get drunk and play silly games—and the party food was delicious. It always seemed like an exciting industry to be part of.

After leaving school, I returned to the industry, working for my uncle in his rapidly expanding empire. He asked me to join him because he could see I found it fascinating. Although I loved the reinvention of the ever-changing clothing trade through fashion and what influenced designers, I also had a passion for homeware and architecture—in fact, I studied architecture through my A levels. I started working in the department store my uncle had just purchased in the Northeast, and at the age of eighteen, I was basically buying for five departments with my cousin, who was not much older than me. Oh, it was so exciting! We would travel to London, Paris and Manchester to fill the store with new ranges that had to be turned around on a two-week basis. I organized adverts, fashion shows and meetings, and I shared the new ranges with all the staff. I worked behind the scenes, but each Saturday I was on the shop floor to see what customers liked and wanted and what we were missing. It reminded me of my parents' store, and I enjoyed the social interaction with customers. Seeing people buying what I had invested in made me smile.

The store was sadly sold, and I was brought into the import side of the business. This was a completely different setup—we were catering to a number of customers at any one time, and we now needed to be ahead of the game, buying for two to three seasons in advance, so my knowledge of fashion, colours and trends was really tested. I still enjoyed it—to be honest, I felt more embedded as I was constantly looking for the newest trends, wanting to mimic what the celebrities and musicians were wearing at that moment in time. I was surely meant to be doing this rather than working with houses, interior design or architecture. Yep, I loved it.

We travelled everywhere—Hong Kong, Shanghai, Guangzhou, Taiwan, Singapore, India, Bangladesh, European cities for the inspiration and New York! I remember going to a Julien Macdonald show during London Fashion Week, and I sat in the front row next to a beautiful lady who was flipping her long, blond hair from side to side and fluttering her eyelashes as the paparazzi flashed constantly. I was in awe and started up a conversation with her. I was always very bold in my approach and didn't have any fear of introducing myself and making friends immediately. As we chatted, it clicked I was sitting next to Jodie Kidd! When the colourful show finished, she stood up, and I came literally up to her waist! It was so embarrassing, so I scurried to the front and tried to peer over everyone to look for other celebrities. That was a moment of sparkle that kept me in the fashion industry. I loved it.

As the years went by and my career took off, I worked my way up to vice president. The family business had been sold to a Hong Kong–based global company. We all still worked there, but there was a change in our attitude towards the business. It shifted from family to corporate, and the pressures of the business were visible on the management team as the industry became tougher and tougher with more competition, new importers, better prices. Whoever had the latest product got the order. Customer loyalty had gone out the window. It was becoming a cutthroat business, now known as 'the rat race'.

I remember going to Tokyo once and seeing these denim styles pulled up like a legging. They were very skinny jeans—at this point (the 2000s), we were all wearing straight leg or carpenter jeans. The skinny jeans looked strange but really cool. I took some back to UK and showed them to my manager. 'We must do these—everyone is wearing them in Tokyo, and they are so comfy.' I was told to buy some more from other influential stores in USA, so we got them and gave them a trial. The jegging sold over two million pieces—it was one of our best sellers, and we did so many different versions for all the retailers. I dedicated a lot of my spare time researching and analyzing the next fashion trends, but it went hand in hand with my interest in homes and social living. I was so interested in the way consumer shopping and living habits were changing. It was something I was really invested in. Seeing the pollution that the industry was causing when I visited cities in the developing world added even more fuel to my natural instinct.

At the beginning of 2014, all managers were given a task to bring something new to the board meeting. I had already been developing a secret range over the previous few weeks, and so I brought in a selection of product—denim, T-shirts, jackets and casual woven wear, all made from recycled, organic or other eco-friendly materials. I presented them, saying, 'This is the future!' I explained how the fashion industry was the second- largest polluter in the world. Everyone looked at me as if I had gone a little crazy and seemed to dismiss the whole idea. I came out deflated but still confident that this was the way to go.

Fast forward to 2020. I took a leap of faith and decided to start my own company and release my own sustainable brands. Sustainable living seemed to be the topic of the moment, and my own eco-friendly brands, which I was very excited and proud to share, were born during COVID-19 lockdown. Reflexone is active-wear made from recycled landfill and ocean plastic, and Ration.L is vegan and gender-neutral trainers and accessories made from recycled, organic and vegan materials.

5 ways you can help improve your carbon footprint through sustainable living:

1. Reduce your meat intake. Have a healthy, balanced diet. Meat production uses high levels of carbon emissions.

2. Reduce using a car. Walk, take public transport or ride a bike. Car emissions are huge contributors to carbon footprint. Otherwise, change it for a greener option.

3. Reduce your energy usage at home. Turn off the lights when not using. Switch off the sockets, TVs, etc. This will reduce your carbon and your bills!

4. Make alternative fashion choices. It's the second-highest pollutant. Buy your things with informed decisions. Wear organic, vegan, recycled, reused.

5. Waste less—this is for all aspects of your home living. Buy only what is needed, not overbuying, and make sustainable choices. Overbuying food, home products and plastics all leads to a high carbon footprint.

Barcode, Reflexone and Ration.L

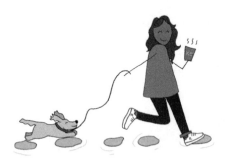

CHAPTER 20

To change your life, you have to change yourself. To change yourself, you have to change your mindset.

—Project Happiness

Yoga and meditation

I TREAT EACH day as my last—not literally, but because I want to enjoy each moment I have and not waste any time. The only way to really experience this moment of pure happiness is to forget yesterday, not think about tomorrow and just indulge in what you are doing this present moment, here and now. After my illness, I had the side effects of short-term memory loss and anxiety over planning what I was going to do in the next few weeks, days, even hours, so I was, in a way, forced to live in the present. I learned this whilst reading one of my favourite books, *I Can See Clearly Now*, by Dr Wayne Dyer. It really taught me to slow down, open my eyes and look around—hear, smell everything surrounding me, as if life were going by in slow motion.

Another tool that has helped me through my anxiety and mental health is meditation. It slows me down and gives me focus on what I am doing at the present moment. I have been practising yoga and meditation for almost ten years now, and it is a routine I can manage and enjoy whilst keeping myself in shape. High-impact cardio raises my blood pressure, which can trigger a seizure—or even worse, another stroke. So I'm happy with doing yoga and feel amazing afterwards. Sometimes I lie on the floor in class while the instructor is talking us through meditation chants, and I just smile and think about how much I'm enjoying this present moment.

I love my walks, and when I go, I notice the simplest things that I never did before. I can see the different colours on the trees, I can smell the leaves and I see the little squirrels scurrying across, collecting things to store. Brandi likes to get a good look too, and sometimes I feel that I have a sort of sixth sense. I notice the smallest detail, sound, smell, image around me as if it's all happening in slow motion. This is something I didn't do before. Whether it was the fast pace of life or the hundreds of tasks I was trying to do on a daily basis, life was just passing by, but what I am experiencing now is just so wonderful.

When I chat with a friend, I like to really listen and understand them instead of thinking about what I'm doing later or if I need to collect some groceries. They appreciate the attention, and I feel that I have been a trusting friend. I like the idea that today is a gift, and we should all embrace it—today is here to be enjoyed because it is the present!

Barcode, Swinging in the park

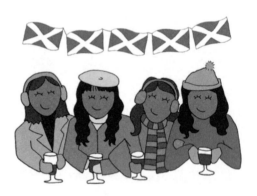

CHAPTER 21

When life gives you lemons, make lemonade!

—ELBERT HUBBARD

IT WAS TIME for a much-needed family bonding trip, and what better place to visit than elegant Edinburgh? And what better time than Christmas? It's a trek, especially from where I live, but we managed to get a forty-minute flight, and it was just perfect. I keep forgetting that Scotland is actually a different country. It seems so near, yet so far.

Anyway, I was excited, my mind filled with anticipation, anxiety and happiness. I wanted to see how Scotland celebrated the holidays—would it live up to our expectations, and what were those, exactly? Since my illness, I actually have *no expectations*, which means that each experience I have is a great big, positive bonus. Anything that gives you happiness when you don't expect it is just pure, undivided joy.

We arrived at the newly renovated Scotsman Hotel and waited patiently for the rest of the family members to arrive. I was ready for some quality time with my dear Jasmine, as she was away at university full-time. With a bluster of footsteps and loud cheering, my sister and her family, my brother and his family and Mummy arrived! We exchanged trip details and checked in. The hotel was very accommodating, putting us all together on the same floor next to each other. The next couple of days were going to be full of fun! We started by taking a brisk walk to see the Christmas markets. It was cold, but as the younger ones settled into the rides, giggling with excitement, the adults headed towards the wooden huts where they were serving mulled wine and hot baked churros. I sat down and smiled. It was lovely to be there, enjoying the moment and spending quality time with my siblings.

After a few more rides and more cheering, we headed for the main shopping street and browsed, then strolled along to Contini, a splendid Italian restaurant on bustling George Street, where we had reservations for our early evening meal. We caught up on what everyone was doing and took turns monitoring the children's table, as Jasmine, now an adult, wanted to join us. When we got back to the hotel, we all changed into our personalized matching pyjamas, ready for games night. The hotel kindly gave us a bar/snug room to enjoy our time together.

Manish, my brother-in-law, was in charge of this event, and we were all given chores for the trip. Mine was to book the hotel, Jasmine and Reena did the itinerary and the Devs were the games masters. What a splendid job they all did! Manish had cleverly incorporated our names into the games, so each question was thoughtful and special and required a very informative answer! It was just perfect. Afterwards, we crashed for a relatively early night, but the children were running room to room, unable to contain the happy energy ☺ of being together.

On Christmas morning, I woke up to a little gift laid next to me. 'I thought we weren't doing gifts to each other this year—I haven't bought you anything', I said with a slightly sad face to my husband.

Deepak replied, 'I'm just saying, you are not the only author in this family!'

I opened the carefully wrapped gift, still in its cardboard mailer.

On the front cover, there were cartoon images of Deepak and me holding hands. The title was *Merry Christmas, Love, Deepak*. The book included many pages of different things he loved about me and a little story of our adventurous life together so far. I could only read a few pages before my eyes started to well up.

'This is the most thoughtful gift I have ever had. Thank you for reminding me who I am and what I mean to you.'

He passed me another book in a similar format, but this was for me to fill in—our adventures ahead, a sort of bucket list of things we could do as a couple and a family. It was so romantic, and I loved it.

Because we were such a large group, the hotel staff served us breakfast in the space they used for wedding parties, but it suited us. We exchanged our secret Santa gifts, and the kids were jumping again. Their eyes lit up as each person opened their gifts.

We had our Christmas meal in the main restaurant area of the hotel. Reena informed me that our table wasn't great for the family, and it would be much better if we were in the comfy booths so we could all talk to each other. As this was the busiest day of the year and only a few hours before dinner, it seemed impossible, but after we all dressed and headed down, the manager, **George Oxley,** kindly made our wish come true! To my dismay, our tables were now number 23 and number 32! Oh, what a wonderful experience it was to spend time with my loved ones over the holidays! This was special and meant to be.

Barcode, The Love Book

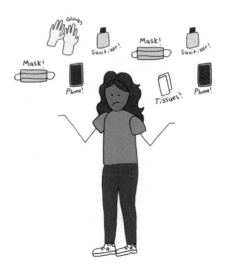

CHAPTER 22

**Our life is shaped by our mind:
we become what we think.**

—GAUTAMA BUDDHA

COVID-19

BEING A BRAIN injury survivor puts me into an extremely vulnerable category. Not because I may catch what is going around quicker—which is also a frightening thought—but because of the anxiety that surrounds it. What if I get ill? What if I go somewhere, and someone there has it and passes it to me? What if I touch something and catch it? What if I don't wash my hands properly? All these what-ifs! Then, even though I have washed my hands thoroughly, I go back and do it again because I've forgotten! Basically, when anything happens, my stress is heightened because of the anxiety that's a side effect of the brain hemorrhage. It just makes me so very nervous. I have said many times that there are levels of brain injury and different spectrums. Many people don't voice what they are thinking, so sometimes I feel a little responsibility to just put it out there.

I was speaking to a friend, explaining what was going through my head in terms of not wanting to go out and finding it difficult when I did go out due to all the questions going around in my head. Her reply was simple: Whether they have a brain injury or not, everyone is actually feeling this way. Well, this just put my mind at ease, because for me, leaving the house is like a military operation:

- ✓ Mask check
- ✓ Hand sanitizer check
- ✓ Gloves check
- ✓ Tissues check
- ✓ Phone check

That's really all you need. But even paying by phone is absolutely stressful. First, you don't know where to find the wallet on your home screen, and then, once you have accomplished that, you can't authorize it because you need to take the mask off because the stupid face ID doesn't work! Anxiety is also worse when wearing a mask. It makes me feel claustrophobic and a little uneasy, so going out wearing a mask for a long period of time is not great for my mental health. I'm looking ahead and trying to let the other person know that I'm smiling at them, but they can't see it.

Anyway, I started to feel that it was too much trouble to go out, so most of the time, I limited my trips and did the things that made me feel comfortable. Going for a walk with family or friends, sitting in my garden or my home, enjoying my surroundings. I will only go to restaurants if I can eat outside. I'm making my own rules! Whether you're a brain injury survivor or not, you need to do things at your pace and comfort level and not get worked up, because it's really not worth it. Surround yourself with people that understand and value your opinions. Life is too short, and it's good to appreciate what you have. Health is wealth, and we are all just trying to adapt to this new normal. Just smile and do what makes you happy!

If you feel what I'm feeling, I would love for you to share this.

5 ways to combat anxiety:

1. Be positive—surround yourself with positive images and people.

2. Be calm—have some downtime and do activities to help reduce anxiety.

3. Be in the present—try not to overload yourself with lists of things to do. Take one step at a time.

4. Be honest—talk to someone if you're feeling overwhelmed.

5. Be happy—all the above will change your mindset to help you towards a happier you!

Barcode, COVID anxiety

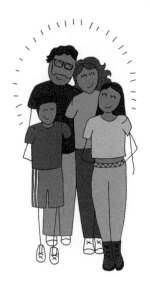

CHAPTER 23

**Life is short, so live it. Love is rare, so
grab it. Memories are precious, so cherish them. We only get one life, so live it!**

—KAVITA BASI

My three Bs

WE ALL KNOW that COVID-19 really changed our society. When
the idea of lockdown came, it created a panic for some and a resting
time for others. I felt right at home already—since my illness, I'd
spent a lot of quality time at home and become used to it. However,
this was lockdown with the family, which was a little stressful but
manageable. We just needed to adjust to this new normal. I focused
for a few months on my three Bs—Brain, Book and Brands!

My brain hemorrhage **still affects my life on a daily basis**—
headaches, tiredness, memory loss and anxiety are just a few of the
lingering effects. So the pandemic has dramatically increased my
anxiety to a point where I can't even look at the news, as it upsets
me—as it may others. I have tried to use that focus and energy to
enjoy my time during lockdown with activities that I really love, like
painting, audiobooks, walking, playing with my dog and resting

to help my anxiety and my **Brain**. It's so, so important to look after your brain and give it some rejuvenating therapy that keeps it stimulated—a little enjoyment turns to happiness. I also thought about how I could reach out to others to share the things that are helping me, so I decided to start a podcast, *Life with No Filter*, with three friends. I feel so proud of this achievement. Here's a link: *https://open.spotify.com/episode/5UCMhohqpwVmWA6ooyRC-JO?si=1m7tZDvYTtiRKzTYH7gEkg.*

My second B is my first Book, *Room 23*, released in November 2018. I can't stress enough how much this book can help others, whether they are in an isolated situation, developed anxiety during lockdown or have mental health issues. I decided to post free copies of my book in the hope that it might give some form of solace to those in need. So off I went on my bike with books wrapped in brown paper in the basket. I dropped off copies to people in my neighbourhood and shared them online with people I thought could really benefit from reading my story—some had an illness or a relative that had recently passed.

In return, I received messages, letters and cards that were so heart-warming I knew it had been the right thing to do. In the meantime, I began work on a new book—the one you are reading right now! **Oh, it's been so therapeutic and lovely to focus on writing**☺**.** If you haven't read *Room 23* yet, please try it☺! Ten percent of the profits of each sale to a great charity, the **Brain & Spine Foundation**. *https://www.amazon.co.uk/Room-23-Surviving-Brain-Hemorrhage/dp/1631524895/ref=tmm_pap_swatch_0?_encoding=UTF8&qid=1607626084&sr=8-1*

Working on **the third B, for Brands,** was very exciting. After over twenty-five years in the fashion industry—during COVID-19, no less—I launched two ethical brands! I think I'm either a little crazy for taking on another task, not that I had enough daily challenges to contend with, or just decided I was going to do it, and whatever happened, happened. I had already spent months in preparation, and the timing felt right, and once they were out, I was excited to see what would be in store for the future. With the disruption in stores, it felt right to have a family business born during a pandemic.

I've always had my heart in protecting our environment, supporting our future generations and looking after our animals, so whilst we had so much time to reflect on, reset and reduce our daily consumption, I released Reflexone and Ration.L. I couldn't do the normal photo shoot with models or a launch party. We were all sticking by the rules and staying home, so we had to be creative in how we showcased the brands. It was hard, with little time for me to even think about the troubles in the world around me. My focus was to try and make the world somehow a better place when the pandemic was all over. Yes, little old me was going to make a difference, if anyone cared to notice. My brands were fashion and accessories made from recycled, organic and vegan materials developed to protect our environment from plastic pollution and landfill. They also give a percentage to the charities I represent in the hope that this would encourage others to buy responsibly.

For several years now, I've bought less and tried to buy ethically, and I think others are now re-evaluating their buying habits after seeing the effects they have had on the beautiful world around us. Climate change has been a message we've been hearing almost every day. I wanted to incorporate what I could into my **brands** to encourage a healthier, happier lifestyle. **Reflexone** activewear is made mostly from recycled, post-industrial plastic, and **Ration.L** is vegan trainers and accessories. They are now available on over eighteen platforms including stores in UK and New York!; you can find out more on the links here:

ReflexOne (@_reflexone) • Instagram photos and videos
RATION.L (@ration.l) • Instagram photos and videos

Barcode, Moments and togetherness

EPILOGUE

I NEVER UNDERSTOOD it when my mum used to say to me, 'Whatever you do in life, never do anything to hurt someone's heart'. Well, not the true meaning of it, anyway. I don't think I was a naturally angry or bad soul at a young age—I don't think anyone is when they are brought into this world. Situations, upbringing and surroundings cause people to change their ways of thinking and being—this is how I see it. No matter how deeply embedded your negativity is, I believe the small steps I share in this book can help lead you towards a better state of mind.

I always like to smile at others, even people I don't know. I believe that when you smile, you create a ripple effect: they smile back, then smile at another person and so on. It's the same with kindness—being kind is a choice, a habit and also a human instinct that should be explored more. I don't think people display enough of it—the selfish emotions always take over. Kindness is helping someone when they need some support; kindness is listening to a close friend. Kindness is giving your child or partner a little pat on the back for doing something well. Kindness is saying thank you. Kindness is being truthful to a friend when they make a mistake, advising them in a soft and gentle manner what they should have done or said.

All of these habits and ways create such a great feeling because the more you practice them, the more they are returned to you in bundles of joy. You, the person displaying kindness, will be happier—go on, try it! Being kind increases those happy endorphins, which, in turn, will bring you a happier, healthier lifestyle.

I have great empathy for others; however, this is something that has scaled up hugely since my illness. My mindset has definitely been focused on these values as a result of my own experiences. One of my friends once said that sometimes a person doesn't have the same empathy because they haven't experienced the same hardship. I think what they were trying to explain is that if a person hasn't lost a close relative or been through a major illness or had major financial issues, then how could they empathise with others who have?

Everyone has their own issues and is going through their own troubles, whether it's not having a matching handbag for the outfit they are wearing, or losing an expensive pair of glasses, or finding out that you only have a few months to live or that someone close to you has a serious illness. You just don't know. When you walk down a street, when you are out shopping, walking through the office at work or even at a school mingling with the other parents, you don't know really what that other person is experiencing, so always go about your day with true kindness. Whoever you meet or speak to, just think about their current situation and show empathy.

DIRECTORY OF USEFUL LINKS

Author | Kavitabasi.com

A World Full of Wonder

Project Happiness

Action for Happiness

Greater Good: The Science of a Meaningful Life (berkeley.edu)

zen habits - breathe zen habits

Gretchen Rubin

Home - Happinez

Practical Happiness Advice That Works | The Positivity Blog

No Sidebar - Design a Simple Life

Spirituality Archives - Change your thoughts (stevenaitchison.co.uk)

Dr Happy | Blog (thehappinessinstitute.com)

mindbodygreen: connecting soul & science

Spiritual Engagement, Meaning and Happiness
(pursuit-of-happiness.org)

9 Keys to Lasting Happiness | Spirituality & Health

Happy Magazines
Happiful Magazine

About us - Breathe (breathemagazine.com)

Planet Mindful magazine (planet-mindful.com)

Live Happy Magazine

Brain, Spine, Mental Health Charities

Generalised anxiety disorder in adults - NHS (www.nhs.uk)

About Anxiety - Anxiety UK

Home | Mind

Brain & Spine Foundation (brainandspine.org.uk)

The Bee Foundation - Brain Aneurysm Research

SameYou

Headway - the brain injury association | Headway

Other Links

ReflexOne (@_reflexone) • Instagram photos and videos

RATION.L (@ration.l) • Instagram photos and videos

http://www.bbc.co.uk/history/people/guy_fawkes

History of Valentine's Day - Facts, Origins & Traditions - HISTORY

https://www.brainandspine.org.uk/about-us/
our-community-ambassadors/

Meet Honey Bash Guest Speaker Kavita Basi - The Bee Foundation

https://www.instagram.com/p/
B08N-KKHT9k/?utm_source=ig_web_copy_link

https://www.amazon.co.uk/Room-23-
Surviving-Brain-Hemorrhage/dp/1631524895/
ref=mp_s_a_1_3?ie=UTF8&qid=1545029421&sr=8-3&pi=AC_SX236_
SY340_QL65&keywords=room+23&dpPl=1&dpID=411TsxkSzSL&ref=plSrch

https://www.kavitabasi.com/publications-1.

http://www.livescience.com/9824-5-happier.html

https://www.thebeefoundation.org/
meet-honey-bash-guest-speaker-kavita-basi/

https://www.anxietyuk.org.uk/anxiety-type/
generalised-anxiety-disorder/?gclid=CjwKCAjw5uTM-
BRAYEiwA5HxQNhtUNhJPa2BkLmSr8o23Ts8B_
DQbeWJozRwOsK8CalKg485oKtoi3BoCQ5UQAvD_BwE

http://www.innerhealthstudio.com/overcoming-anxiety.html

YouTube: https://www.youtube.com/watch?v=NT3lR9ss36E

IGTV: https://www.instagram.com/tv/B-q9_4Fnvys/

https://www.corraldelrey.com/corral-del-rey

https://open.spotify.com/episode/5UCMhohqpwVm-
WA6ooyRCJO?si=1m7tZDvYTtiRKzTYH7gEkg

https://www.amazon.co.uk/Room-23-Surviving-Brain-Hemorrhage/
dp/1631524895/ref=tmm_pap_swatch_0?_encod-
ing=UTF8&qid=1607626084&sr=8-1

Would love to connect with you!

If you want a little motivation or like to get
some positive vibes, please follow me on

Instagram @kavita_basi

Twitter @KavitaBasi

Facebook @KavitaBasiroom23

Otherwise, you can email me or follow my
blog on www.kavitabasi.com.

Printed in Great Britain
by Amazon

25843591R00079